Occupational Therapy in Action

A LIBRARY OF CASE STUDIES

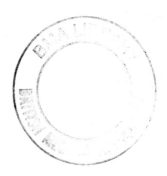

Occupational Therapy in Action

A LIBRARY OF CASE STUDIES

Dianne Trickey-Rokenbrod, OTD, MBA, OTR/L

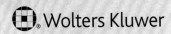

Philadelphia • Baltimore • New York • London
Buenos Aires • Hong Kong • Sydney • Tokyo

Acquisitions Editor: Michael Nobel
Product Development Editor: Linda Francis
Editorial Assistant: Tish Rogers
Marketing Manager: Shauna Kelley
Production Project Manager: David Orzechowski
Design Coordinator: Stephen Druding
Artist/Illustrator: Christine Mercer-Vernon
Manufacturing Coordinator: Margie Orzech
Prepress Vendor: S4Carlisle Publishing Services

First Edition

9 8 7 6 5 4 3 2 1

Printed in China

Library of Congress Cataloging-in-Publication Data

Trickey-Rokenbrod, Dianne, author.
  Occupational therapy in action : a library of case studies / Dianne Trickey-Rokenbrod.
  p. ; cm.
  Includes bibliographical references and index.
  ISBN 978-1-4963-1028-6
  I. Title.
  [DNLM: 1. Occupational Therapy—Case Reports. 2. Decision Making—Case Reports. WB 555]
  RM735
  615.8'515—dc23
                                                                        2015035903

LWW.com

This book is dedicated to the many people I have worked with as clients over the course of 30-plus years as an occupational therapist. I thank you for your generosity in sharing your life stories, which have been woven into the spirit of these cases. To my students, whose desire to help others gave rise to this manual: you continue to intrigue and challenge me. And to my husband, Bill, and my daughters, Alicia, Kendra, and Erica: you are my inspiration and joy always.

Reviewers

Carla Chase, EdD, OTR/L
Associate Professor
Department of Occupational Therapy
Western Michigan University
Kalamazoo, Michigan

Wanda I. Colon, PhD, OTR/L
OT Program Director, Associate Professor
Department of Occupational Therapy
University of Puerto Rico, Medical Sciences
  Campus
San Juan, Puerto Rico

Kari C. Inda, PhD, OTR
Chairperson, Associate Professor
Department of Occupational Therapy
Mount Mary University
Milwaukee, Wisconsin

Debra Lindstrom, PhD, OTR/L
Professor
Department of Occupational Therapy
Western Michigan University
Kalamazoo, Michigan

Cathy M. Mistovich, MS, OTR/L
Program Director-OTA/Department Chair-Health
  Professions
Department of Health Professions/OTA
South Suburban College
South Holland, Illinois

Toni S. Oakes, EdD, MS, OTR/L
OT Program Director
School of Occupational Therapy
Lenoir-Rhyne University
Hickory, North Carolina

Dawndra M. Sechrist, OTR, PhD
Program Director
Department of Rehabilitation Sciences
Master of Occupational Therapy Program
Texas Tech University Health Sciences Center
Lubbock, Texas

Jeanine Stancanelli, OTD, MPH, OTR/L
Associate Professor and Interim Associate
  Director
Department of Occupational Therapy
Dobbs Ferry, New York

Christine Vicino, MA, OTA/L
Program Director
Department of Occupational Therapy
Grossmont College
El Cajon, California

About the Author

Dianne Trickey-Rokenbrod, OTD, MBA, OTR/L, is currently Chair and Associate Professor of the Occupational Therapy Division at Keuka College in New York. This rather recent adventure follows a career that includes over thirty years of working with clients in both residential and community settings, managing rehabilitation programs, helping to build and operate nursing homes, and management consulting. The common denominator continues to be helping people achieve a fulfilling life. Dianne and her husband Bill live in the rural hills of Western New York when they are not sailing the Eastern Seaboard on *Tres Hijas*.

Preface

Occupational Therapy in Action: A Library of Case Studies is designed for students who have already learned the basic tools for assessing and treating commonly seen conditions in occupational therapy and who are ready to integrate and apply their knowledge. With the variety of practice settings in today's healthcare system, occupational therapists must be prepared to make numerous treatment decisions every day—but teaching students *how* to make those decisions is a very different challenge from teaching them concepts or showing them what to do in a lab. The purpose of this book is to teach both the *why* and the *how* of making decisions in actual client treatment sessions. It does so by helping students hone and apply their clinical and professional reasoning skills in a logical, step-by-step process that can be replicated in any case, in any setting. The Case Development Protocol detailed in Chapter 2 is that process, and it was developed and refined through my own teaching experience.

Depending on instructor preference, this manual may be used either at the end of a unit of study, to help students integrate their learning by working with cases that correspond to the conditions studied, or as the foundation for an advanced course designed to challenge students to apply their learning across a broad spectrum of conditions. For curricula that are organized around the continuum of care, an Index of Conditions by Practice Setting is available to facilitate the sequencing of material (see Appendix C).

The cases themselves contain information and details that are designed to create a realistic experience of working with actual client cases. They contain references to common medications, typical complications, and personal conflicts, along with descriptions of medical, nursing, and other aspects of care that reflect the complexity of clients' lives in a variety of treatment settings. The terms *patient*, *client*, *resident*, and *participant* are used as appropriate to the setting depicted, with an awareness that some agencies are working to change the image that certain terms may evoke. It is not my intention to perpetuate any negative image through the use of these terms. All cases are original and were designed specifically for this manual; any resemblance to actual people is purely coincidental.

Approach

The effectiveness of case-based teaching methods is well established. Case studies as teaching tools offer significant psychological, social, and intellectual dimensions, and working through them offers students the opportunity to exercise higher-level cognitive skills and complex reasoning. Cases also provide exposure to different settings, diagnoses, and contexts that can help students learn to apply their knowledge more easily when they encounter unfamiliar situations. Such practice increases their self-confidence and helps prepare them for situations in which they must independently plan appropriate assessments and interventions in actual cases.

This book evolved out of my efforts to help students learn to apply the information from their previous coursework to hands-on client treatment. The approach presented in this manual, the core of which is the Case Development Protocol, grew out of my own experience in teaching the material for a course based originally on Dr. Vicki Smith's book *Occupational Therapy: Transition From Classroom to Clinic—Physical Disability Fieldwork Applications* (1994). Other works that influenced my own development include Fleming and Mattingly's *Clinical Reasoning: Forms of Inquiry in a Therapeutic Practice* (1994), Schell and Schell's *Clinical and Professional Reasoning in Occupational Therapy* (2008), and Fink's *Creating Significant Learning Experiences* (2003). The assignments and teaching techniques suggested in this manual also reflect insights that came from many discussions with colleagues to tease out effective methods of developing students' reasoning skills.

The Case Development Protocol itself is a unique step-by-step process that teaches occupational therapy students to apply clinical reasoning to the analysis and planning of initial treatment sessions. Each step in developing the case is intentional, requiring reflection and purposeful, informed choices. Although breaking down the process into so many steps initially might seem time-consuming, it is an essential part of helping students develop clinical reasoning. Like any other skill, clinical reasoning must be broken down into its component parts and practiced in a systematic way before it becomes instinctive. The Case Development Protocol is designed to be used with the sample cases in Part II as preparation for practice in actual treatment settings.

Organization

This book is arranged in two parts:

- **Part I, Foundations of Occupational Therapy Practice,** describes how your knowledge of theory and clinical reasoning guide treatment decisions that you will make throughout your practice (Chapter 1) as well as a step-by-step approach to working through a typical case (Chapter 2).
- **Part II, Practice Cases,** includes musculoskeletal cases (Chapter 3), neurologic cases (Chapter 4), cardiopulmonary cases (Chapter 5), organ system cases (Chapter 6), and mental disorder cases (Chapter 7), in a variety of treatment settings. Chapter 8 offers a selection of interprofessional cases to aid in the development of interprofessional skills.

Chapter 1, "Informed Clinical Choices: Conceptual Practice Models and Clinical Reasoning," summarizes relevant conceptual practice models, explores how the choice of practice model affects the occupational therapist's clinical choices, and discusses six common types of clinical reasoning, with examples of types of decisions made using each. The combination of sound theory and logical choices based on an understanding of clinical reasoning is designed to help students apply their knowledge of assessment and intervention safely, efficiently, and effectively.

Chapter 2, "Case Development Protocol," focuses on the method that students will use to develop the practice cases in Part II. This chapter offers a detailed demonstration of how each step of the Protocol may be applied to a sample case. Before students start using the Protocol with the practice cases, they should complete the Student Skills Survey in Appendix A. The results of this survey will indicate the areas on which they most need to focus.

In Part II, **Chapters 3 through 7** are grouped by diagnostic category. The introduction to Part II includes a detailed table titled "Practice Cases: Clients, Conditions, and Care Settings" that serves as an index to all the cases. The information it provides about clients' conditions and the care settings covered will be useful in helping students focus their work on specific areas. The clients depicted in the sample cases display unique individual characteristics that will provide rich, realistic personal context. Each sample case is presented chronologically, as if the student is reading a client's chart to gather background information and then meeting the client for the first time. Each case description takes students up to the point at which occupational therapy treatment is about to begin. Some cases follow a client into a second setting along the continuum of care, with similar information given for the second setting. The result is a comprehensive case study that calls upon students to demonstrate clinical reasoning throughout.

Chapter 8, "Interprofessional Cases," reflects the evolving trend in health care toward providers sharing joint responsibility for outcomes of care. As research and public policy continue to shape practice, it becomes increasingly important for practitioners in the individual health professions to receive interactive, experiential interprofessional education. The cases in this chapter are designed to provide just such a learning experience by fostering discussion among students in different disciplines. Although the disciplines involved in a discussion will naturally vary depending on the programs available at a particular institution, the same overall process may be applied in any interprofessional case, with the assessments and interventions discussed and developed collaboratively, with contributions from the unique perspective of each of the different disciplines.

The **Appendices** provide not only the Student Skills Assessment and Index of Practice Settings (Appendices A and C, respectively) but also a detailed version of the complete Case Development Protocol (Appendix B), an Occupational Therapy Practice Framework Worksheet (Appendix D), and a variety of forms (Appendix E) that students will use in developing their practice cases. Students may find it especially useful to photocopy Appendix B and keep a copy of the Case Development Protocol close at hand for reference when working through the steps in each practice case.

The User's Guide that follows provides a detailed look at the unique pedagogical features included in this book, and describes how each one contributes to the learning process.

Online Resources

Instructors will find a variety of resources available at http://thePoint.lww.com to help get the most out of this text:

- Video demonstrations by students working through the cases
- A case-based teaching overview that provides helpful tips
- A case development scoring rubric
- Instructions for "Grand Rounds," a learning exercise developed by the author
- Instructions for working with interprofessional case development
- PowerPoints

Students will find a variety of blank forms for printing out and using, in their study and practice.

Acknowledgments

I want to acknowledge my academic mentor and colleague, Vicki Smith, EdD, OTR/L, FAOTA, whose book *Occupational Therapy: Transition From Classroom to Clinic—Physical Disability Fieldwork Applications* (American Occupational Therapy Association, 1994) is part of this book's foundation. It was with Smith's encouragement that I took over instruction of a capstone occupational therapy course at Keuka College that had originally been based in part on her book. That experience taught me how to help students develop the clinical reasoning to apply the knowledge already learned in their previous coursework.

For assistance during the development of this manual, I also want to recognize my wonderful friend Jo-Anne Taylor, BSN, for medication recommendations and other medical content; my daughter Alicia Manktelow, BSN, for critical care review, and my colleagues Christopher Alterio, Dr. OT, OTR/L, Cassie Hay, OTR/L, and Sunny Winstead, OTR/L, for reviewing select cases in their respective areas of expertise. At the same time, I take sole responsibility for any errors in this manual.

Finally, this book would never have been published without the encouragement of Michael Nobel, Executive Editor at Wolters Kluwer, and the wonderful team he brought on board to nurture and refine my efforts, specifically, Linda Francis and Dana Knighten.

—Dianne Trickey-Rokenbrod

User's Guide

In today's evolving healthcare environment, it's more important than ever that you be thoroughly prepared to work with a variety of clients in a variety of practice settings, and that you know how to do so collaboratively, sharing accountability for outcomes with healthcare professionals from many other disciplines. You will need strong clinical reasoning skills to help you plan assessments and interventions that will enable you to deliver safe, effective care to your clients. Seasoned occupational therapists make logical clinical decisions in a fluid way that makes it seem almost instinctive. But how can you develop and practice your clinical reasoning skills before you actually start treating patients? This book is designed to help you do just that.

Clinical reasoning is a learned skill that can be broken down into individual steps and honed through systematic, repetitive practice. **Part I** of this book provides the background information you'll need as preparation, and **Part II** offers the "hands-on" practice.

- **Chapter 1** compares various conceptual practice models and compares six types of clinical reasoning.
- **Chapter 2** then teaches you the step-by-step process—the Case Development Protocol—that you will use to work with the practice cases in Part II. As you progress through Chapter 2, you will be asked to consider the impact that specific context has on your clinical decisions. Each step in the Case Development Protocol presents opportunities for you to apply different methods of clinical reasoning to help you develop and adjust treatment for your unique "client."

Developing clinical reasoning requires a different kind of learning from any you may have encountered so far. By working with the realistic case studies in Part II, you will be challenged to analyze thoughtfully both *what* decisions you need to make and *how* you will make them. You will use the Case Development Protocol to develop a case, starting with the initial referral and introduction to your new "client," proceeding through the assessment process, and finishing with development of an intervention plan as well as a plan for the first five treatment sessions. You will also consider home programs, discharge planning, and effective collaboration with assistants and other team members.

As you work through the practice cases, you will come to "know" some of the characters as if they were truly your clients. Just as you would with real clients, you will spend time thinking about the clients' lives and challenges, modifying your plans and the details of how you plan to help them reach their goals. Your efforts to develop your clinical reasoning skills now will be rewarded by the impact you will have on the lives you will touch in the future.

(continues on page xviii)

Features

This User's Guide introduces you to the special tools in this book that will enhance your learning experience.

A. Overall, how well prepared do you feel right now to evaluate and treat clients with typical diagnoses that you have studied?

    1   2   3   4   5   6   7   8   9   10

I would not be capable of   *I feel very confident that I could*
providing any effective OT   *provide effective OT*
evaluation or treatment   *evaluation and treatment*

B. Please enter a score between 1 (very low) and 10 (very high) for each category below that reflects your perception of your ability to successfully identify and administer assessments and interventions for clients with typical diagnoses.

1. Traumatic and repetitive stress musculoskeletal conditions
   (e.g., carpal tunnel syndrome, arm fractures, tendon repairs) _____
2. Chronic musculoskeletal conditions (e.g., rheumatoid arthritis) _____
3. Traumatic neurological injuries (e.g., cerebral vascular accident, spinal cord injury) _____
4. Progressive neurological conditions (e.g., multiple sclerosis, dementia) _____
5. Cardiopulmonary conditions
   (e.g., myocardial infarction, chronic obstructive pulmonary disease) _____
6. Organ system conditions (e.g., burns, diabetes, cancer) _____
7. Mental disorders (e.g., major depression, schizophrenia) _____

C. Why do you think your highest scores above are this high?

The **Student Skills Assessment** evaluates your readiness to start providing care for a variety of conditions in diverse practice settings. **Reflection questions** help you identify areas where you need more practice, allowing you to create a targeted development plan.

Step 1. What demographic information do I have for my client?

1. Review your case and list the basic demographic information.
2. What other basic information do you need that is not in the case description? What other source(s) might supply this information?

Step 2. What information can I find about my client's primary condition?

1. Review your case and document the primary condition or diagnosis you will be treating. Include any mention of symptoms, and any objective data about the condition or diagnosis.
2. Is all of the information you found relevant to your occupational therapy treatment? Explain your answer.
3. What type(s) of clinical reasoning did you use to guide your answer to question 2?

Step 3. Does my client have any secondary conditions?

1. Review your case and identify any secondary conditions, complications, or

The **Case Development Protocol** is the step-by-step process you'll use to practice applying your clinical and professional reasoning skills in the practice cases. Following this logical and sequential process will hone your clinical reasoning skills and prepare you to develop cases in multiple practice settings.

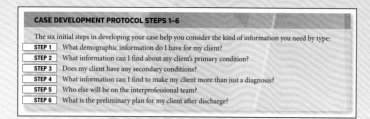

CASE DEVELOPMENT PROTOCOL STEPS 1–6

The six initial steps in developing your case help you consider the kind of information you need by type:

STEP 1   What demographic information do I have for my client?
STEP 2   What information can I find about my client's primary condition?
STEP 3   Does my client have any secondary conditions?
STEP 4   What information can I find to make my client more than just a diagnosis?
STEP 5   Who else will be on the interprofessional team?
STEP 6   What is the preliminary plan for my client after discharge?

Case Development Protocol Boxes appear with chapter headings and list all the main Case Development Protocol questions discussed in that section. These boxes help you quickly locate material related to particular Protocol steps, serving as a handy aid as you work through the cases.

Developing Your Case | STEP 2

What information can I find about my client's primary condition?

1. Review your case and document the primary condition or diagnosis you will be treating. Include any mention of symptoms, and any objective data about the condition or diagnosis.

2. Is all of the information you found relevant to your occupational therapy treatment? Explain your answer.

3. What type(s) of clinical reasoning did you use to guide your answer to question 2?

Developing Your Case: Step by Step boxes spotlight each individual step in the Case Development Protocol. They offer more detail than the Case Development Protocol boxes, by including both the main question in the step and any related subquestions. These boxes will guide your thinking as you develop the clinical reasoning at each step.

Sample forms are included to help you work through some of the steps in the Case Development Protocol. Some of the figures in Chapter 2 depict parts of these forms with sample responses completed. Blank versions of the forms are provided in the Appendices.

5-DAY TREATMENT SESSION PLANNING FORM

Patient Name: _Angela X._

Day 1 1.5 hours total	Day 2 1.5 hours total	Day 3 1.5 hours total	Day 4 1.5 hours total	Day 5 1.5 hours total
Assessments: *COPM* .5 hr *MMT BUE and dynamometer* .5 hr *Start SCIM* .5 hr	Assessments: *Finish SCIM* .5 hr	Assessments:	Assessments: *Give Interest Checklist to complete on own.*	Assessments:
Interventions:	Interventions:	Interventions:	Interventions:	Interventions:
Plan: *Finish initial assessments.*	Plan: *Create intervention plan.*	Plan:	Plan:	Plan: *Reassess MMT, dynamometer, and SCIM.*
HP:	HP:	HP:	HP:	HP:

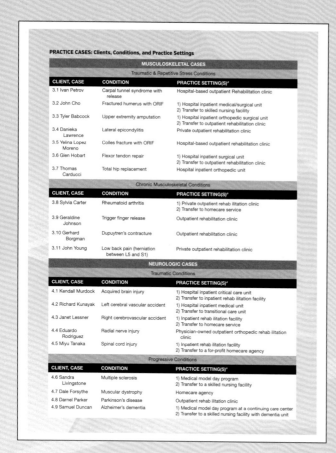

PRACTICE CASES: Clients, Conditions, and Practice Settings

MUSCULOSKELETAL CASES		
Traumatic & Repetitive Stress Conditions		
CLIENT, CASE	**CONDITION**	**PRACTICE SETTING(S)ª**
3.1 Ivan Petrov	Carpal tunnel syndrome with release	Hospital-based outpatient Rehabilitation clinic
3.2 John Cho	Fractured humerus with ORIF	1) Hospital inpatient medical/surgical unit 2) Transfer to skilled nursing facility
3.3 Tyler Babcock	Upper extremity amputation	1) Hospital inpatient orthopedic surgical unit 2) Transfer to outpatient rehabilitation clinic
3.4 Danieka Lawrence	Lateral epicondylitis	Private outpatient rehabilitation clinic
3.5 Yelina Lopez Moreno	Colles fracture with ORIF	Hospital-based outpatient rehabilitation clinic
3.6 Glen Hobart	Flexor tendon repair	1) Hospital inpatient surgical unit 2) Transfer to outpatient rehabilitation clinic
3.7 Thomas Carducci	Total hip replacement	Hospital inpatient orthopedic unit
Chronic Musculoskeletal Conditions		
CLIENT, CASE	**CONDITION**	**PRACTICE SETTING(S)ª**
3.8 Sylvia Carter	Rheumatoid arthritis	1) Private outpatient rehabilitation clinic 2) Transfer to homecare service
3.9 Geraldine Johnson	Trigger finger release	Outpatient rehabilitation clinic
3.10 Gerhard Borgman	Dupuytren's contracture	Outpatient rehabilitation clinic
3.11 John Young	Low back pain (herniation between L5 and S1)	Private outpatient rehabilitation clinic
NEUROLOGIC CASES		
Traumatic Conditions		
CLIENT, CASE	**CONDITION**	**PRACTICE SETTING(S)ª**
4.1 Kendall Murdock	Acquired brain injury	1) Hospital inpatient critical care unit 2) Transfer to inpatient rehabilitation facility
4.2 Richard Kunayak	Left cerebral vascular accident	1) Hospital inpatient medical unit 2) Transfer to transitional care unit
4.3 Janet Lessner	Right cerebrovascular accident	1) Inpatient rehabilitation facility 2) Transfer to homecare service
4.4 Eduardo Rodriguez	Radial nerve injury	Physician-owned outpatient orthopedic rehabilitation clinic
4.5 Miyu Tanaka	Spinal cord injury	1) Inpatient rehabilitation facility 2) Transfer to a for-profit homecare agency
Progressive Conditions		
CLIENT, CASE	**CONDITION**	**PRACTICE SETTING(S)ª**
4.6 Sandra Livingstone	Multiple sclerosis	1) Medical model day program 2) Transfer to a skilled nursing facility
4.7 Dale Forsythe	Muscular dystrophy	Homecare agency
4.8 Darnel Parker	Parkinson's disease	Outpatient rehabilitation clinic
4.9 Samuel Duncan	Alzheimer's dementia	1) Medical model day program at a continuing care center 2) Transfer to a skilled nursing facility with dementia unit

Part II's introduction includes an index to all the sample cases, titled **Practice Cases: Clients, Conditions, and Care Settings**. This table provides a quick summary that helps you find cases that center around a particular condition or take place in a particular setting—so you can quickly locate the cases that correspond to the areas you most need to develop.

Case Notes boxes appear at the beginning of each practice case in Part II. They list the client's name, the condition for which he or she is being treated, and the setting.

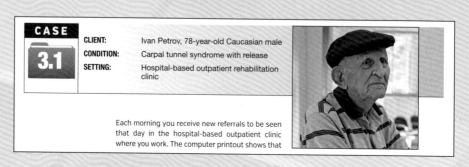

CASE 3.1

CLIENT:	Ivan Petrov, 78-year-old Caucasian male
CONDITION:	Carpal tunnel syndrome with release
SETTING:	Hospital-based outpatient rehabilitation clinic

Each morning you receive new referrals to be seen that day in the hospital-based outpatient clinic where you work. The computer printout shows that

Questions as You Begin

Consider these questions as you begin developing this c

- How much strength and coordination will Mr. Petrov r doing the work on the farm?
- Are there other meaningful roles that he could transiti over more of his physical chores?
- What will happen as they age?
- Should you ask these questions, or is it outside of the sc

Questions as You Begin boxes appear at the end of every case. These are case-specific questions to consider at the outset of your work. They are designed to develop your awareness of and insight into factors that influence your client and his or her response to treatment that could be overlooked at the very beginning of treatment. Answering them thoughtfully will help hone your interpersonal skills and help you develop strong therapeutic relationships.

Contents

Foundations of Occupational Therapy Practice

This foundational portion of the book contains a chapter describing how your knowledge of theory and clinical reasoning guide occupational therapy practice. This is followed by the Case Development Protocol, a step-by-step approach to working through a typical case. Part II gives you an opportunity to apply this process to a wide range of cases in a variety of practice settings.

Informed Clinical Choices: Conceptual Practice Models and Clinical Reasoning

It has been said that occupational therapy students develop clinical reasoning only with the experience of working directly with clients in treatment settings. Even when you are working in a treatment setting under clinical supervision, though, your clinical supervisor probably will not address the process of clinical reasoning early in your training. Good clinical supervisors will certainly model clinical reasoning for you, but their discussions and teaching will likely center around helping you perfect your clinical technique, treatment planning, and documentation and learning to work effectively in an interprofessional team environment.

Clinical reasoning is a cornerstone of effective occupational therapy practice. It is not a skill that develops passively or spontaneously—but it is a skill you can start developing even before you begin working directly with clients. Having solid clinical reasoning skills before doing hands-on treatment can not only help increase your self-confidence and decrease your anxiety but can also lessen potential frustration for both you and your clinical supervisor.

The term *professional reasoning* is sometimes used instead of *clinical reasoning* to reflect the fact that occupational therapists provide treatment in a variety of settings, not just clinical or medical settings. This book uses the more common term *clinical reasoning* to refer to all decisions that occupational therapy practitioners make that directly or indirectly affect client care, regardless of practice setting. This broader concept of clinical reasoning is best defined as "the process that practitioners use to plan, direct, perform, and reflect on client care."[1]

This book is designed to help you learn how and why clinical decisions are made and to give you an opportunity to build your clinical reasoning skills by working through realistic client cases. Part I focuses on the theoretical underpinnings of practice: how the choice of conceptual practice model and the use of different types of clinical reasoning guide your clinical choices. Chapter 2 presents a step-by-step process to help you learn to develop a case, making realistic clinical decisions on how to approach, assess and treat an assigned client. Before you begin working through a case from Part II, your instructor might have you complete the Student Skills Survey in Appendix A. The results of this survey will give you and your instructor a sense of the areas where you most need to focus your efforts.

THE CASE DEVELOPMENT PROCESS: A SUMMARY

Identifying Relevant Information in the Record

1. Demographic information

2. Primary condition

3. Secondary conditions

4. Personal context

5. Interprofessional team

6. Preliminary discharge plan

Developing the Occupational Profile

7. Draft interview questions

8. Occupational profile

9. Implications for treatment

Preparing for Evidence-Based Practice

10. Evidence-based review

Projecting the Impact of the Condition on Performance

11. Impact of primary and secondary conditions on performance

Setting as Context

12. Characteristics of the treatment environment

13. Length of treatment

14. Occupational therapist's role on the interprofessional team

Assessment

15. Specific assessment tools for evaluating your client

16. Your client's assessment results

Creating the Intervention Plan

17. Beginning an intervention plan

18. Occupational performance deficits (areas of focus in treatment)

19. Client's strengths

20. Occupational performance goals

21. Types of interventions

22. Frequency of treatments

Planning the First Five Treatment Sessions

23. Organization of sessions

Planning a Home Program

24. Tailoring the program to support client progress

Daily Treatment Documentation

25. Communicating daily treatment activity

Creating a Discharge Plan

26. Considering client needs

Coordinating and Delegating Care

27. Coordinating with an occupational therapy assistant

Ethics in Practice

28. Considering ethical dilemmas

Therapeutic Use of Self, the OTPF-III, and Clinical Reasoning

Occupational therapists today practice within the paradigm of the American Occupational Therapy Association's (AOTA) Occupational Therapy Practice Framework, which is now in its third edition (hereafter abbreviated OTPF-III).[2] This document describes, defines, and guides the practice of occupational therapy, outlining both the responsibilities of the job and its unique contributions to health promotion. The OTPF-III uses the term *therapeutic use of self* (TUOS) to refer to the process by which occupational therapists establish and maintain the therapeutic relationship with clients. TUOS is an integral part of the occupational therapy process as described by OTPF-III.

Just as TUOS is integral to the occupational therapy process as a whole, so too clinical reasoning is integral to both TUOS and the occupational therapy (OT) process. Clinical reasoning can be described as the bridge between the knowledge obtained in the classroom and treatment of a real client. Clinical reasoning is the process by which therapists use their knowledge to make the myriad decisions every day that result in the therapeutic relationships and activities known as occupational therapy. The OTPF-III embraces Taylor & Van Puymbroecks' philosophy that describes three different approaches the occupational therapist uses to develop intentional relationships with clients by means of TUOS: empathy, client-centered collaboration, and narrative and clinical reasoning.[3] The final section of this chapter focuses on the latter by exploring six of the most recognized types of clinical reasoning.

Conceptual Practice Models

It may seem as if theory is left in the classroom once hands-on work in a clinic or other practice setting begins. Although therapists do not typically talk about and document the theory or paradigm used to treat each client, their clinical choices, nevertheless, are very much guided by the various theoretical "lenses" through which they view the client and the therapy process. Occupational therapy researcher Gary Kielhofner explains these lenses thus: "Conceptual practice models provide special professional lenses through which the therapist sees the client and the therapy process, develops plans, and solves problems."[4] This book uses Kielhofner's broader term *conceptual practice model* rather than the more limited terms *theory* and *frame of reference*.

As Kielhofner explains, a conceptual practice model includes theory, practice resources, and evidence that demonstrate how the model works within the unique occupational therapy paradigm. Kielhofner's book *Conceptual Foundations of Occupational Therapy Practice* explores a variety of the most common occupational therapy conceptual practice models. Some of these models, such as the biomechanical model, have been in use for many years, whereas others, such as the motor control model, are more recent.

Under the OTPF-III umbrella, a conceptual practice model is used to guide the occupational therapist's practice. Conceptual practice models can encourage sound clinical decision making about such things as prioritizing time spent with clients and the choice of assessments and interventions used. The choice of appropriate conceptual practice model varies. Factors that influence this choice include the setting or practice environment, the client's diagnosis or condition, and the occupational therapist's training and knowledge, among others. A comparison of the older biomechanical model with a second model reveals the impact this choice can have on treatment decisions.

Two Conceptual Practice Models Compared

A comparison of two models will be used to illustrate the impact this clinical choice has on practice.

Biomechanical Model

The biomechanical model has a long history in occupational therapy practice, particularly in traditional medical settings, and according to the National Board for Certification in Occupational Therapy,[5] it is still widely used. As occupational therapy's emphasis on client-centered care and occupational performance has re-emerged as being central to the practice of OT, however, the discipline has steadily moved away from the medical model of care.[6] With this in mind, let us consider a practice setting of an acute medical hospital with a rehabilitation department staffed by occupational and physical therapists.

The medical hospital's rehabilitation clinic has a lot of gym equipment along with many different preparatory modalities, some fine motor and perceptual training tools, and the usual assortment of treatment tables and divided treatment spaces. The occupational therapist's treatment space does not include a kitchen or bathroom. Most of the clients treated in this clinic have symptoms related to musculoskeletal conditions, except for the occasional client with a neurological diagnosis.

The occupational therapist in this example bases his or her practice primarily on the biomechanical conceptual practice model, which guides the therapist to focus assessments primarily on deficits in musculoskeletal deficits and their underlying causes—for example, assessment of strength, range of motion, and sensory deficits. The therapist's interventions are focused on reducing these deficits and addressing the underlying client factors with the aim of maintaining or restoring occupational performance.[7] All too often, the interventions in this setting use the often-seen stacking cones, therapy putty, and pinch pins. If the therapist is creative, he or she may manage to make the sessions more motivating by bringing in objects to use in familiar activities, such as games or crafts. Even so, the therapist chooses interventions based on the client's deficit area and grades the interventions carefully to increase the challenge as the client's tolerance or capacity increases. Progress is measured through improvement of the deficit areas.

In the vocabulary of OTPF-III, the approach in the biomechanical conceptual practice model would be described as addressing client factors of body function and structure, the reasoning being that as these underlying client factors improve, the therapist moves on to help the client regain performance skills. Activities and equipment are modified to close the gap between the client's capacities and the task demands of desired performance skills. Occupation is used to provide meaning and motivation, but the focus remains on reducing underlying deficits.

Basing practice on this model results in a narrow, "bottom-up" approach to treatment whose desired goal is the client's achieving occupational performance goals through improved individual client factors. The term *bottom-up* refers to the starting point, which is the examination and treatment of the underlying building blocks that cause performance deficits.

The focus of the biomechanical model is narrow as opposed to holistic and can lead the therapist to overlook important issues. The concern in choosing to be guided only by this model is that it severely limits not only the therapist's intervention choices but also the client's role in the process. Because early treatments aimed at regaining strength, mobility, and endurance often are not occupation-based, they are less engaging for the client and do not carry over as well in the client's natural environment. The client's role in the process is passive with minimal client choice, unlike the central role that OTPF-III describes for the client in therapy, in which the client is actively engaged in guiding treatments selected to achieve his or her own future life goals. As the discipline of occupational therapy continues to evolve, the biomechanical model, although still recognized professionally, is becoming less compatible with the new, more client-centered paradigm.

Occupational Adaptation Practice Model

In contrast, consider the occupational adaptation practice model developed by Schkade and Schultz,[8] and how it plays out in the course of a client's treatment. A personal example will illustrate.

For several years, I worked in an acute rehabilitation setting similar to the medical setting described above. As healthcare reimbursement practices changed, my patients stayed for shorter and shorter periods of time, and I struggled to make the best use of my limited time with them. I finally decided that the most effective approach would be to teach them to become "their own best therapists"—that is, to be prepared to return home, my clients would need to develop their own personal ability to problem solve and adapt to occupations in a different environment. No matter how sophisticated my equipment and space were in the clinic, they were never going to be like my clients' homes. And once my clients left the rehabilitation setting, I would not be there to help them.

I had learned about the occupational adaptation practice model and its emphasis on the innate drive that each person has to achieve relative mastery of valued occupations. According to Schkade and Schultz, occupational adaptation occurs as a natural process when individuals are engaged in a valued occupation and need to find ways to adapt through active problem solving, but this natural ability can become overwhelmed by impairment, illness, or other stressors. In this model, the goal of therapy is to maximize the individual's ability to adapt to his or her unique challenges in order to achieve satisfactory performance of desired occupations. Interventions are chosen based on their capacity to support the client's internal adaptation process by helping them cope with and adapt to the challenges presented by an injury or illness.

Using this practice model, I chose activities that simulated the occupations my clients most wanted to resume engaging in, and I helped them problem solve using either the actual occupation or a situation that resembled it as closely as the setting would allow. I took the time to discuss activity analysis or adaptations for my clients' particular conditions so that they could use the same techniques I had learned. I also assigned outside work that included problem solving on the client's own time, to build their skills and improve performance.

My clinical decisions about assessments also evolved under this practice model. I began using the Canadian Occupational Performance Measure[9] to identify the occupations my clients were most motivated to work on, and we chose interventions based on it. My clients took the lead on problem solving, and home programs became challenges to apply what we had discovered in treatment to other occupations they were interested in. Now the focus was "top down"—starting with the big picture of what my clients wanted to be able to do and proceeding from that point. This was a much more holistic and client-centered view.

Comparing these two different practice models in similar settings demonstrates how a practice model and its underlying theory can affect the occupational therapist's clinical decisions. As this comparison also implies, all practice models have their own limitations and benefits that must be considered thoughtfully. As you become more familiar with different models through your study, fieldwork, and hands-on experience, you will develop more facility in using them to address different situations. The client who has both physical and mental dysfunctions may challenge you to use more than one practice model in treating the same person! In every case, it is important to be thoughtful and purposeful when choosing a conceptual practice model, because that choice guides your clinical choices, and those in turn affect your clients and their success in achieving their goals. As you analyze and develop the practice cases in this book, you will have an opportunity to discuss the practice model and theoretical support underlying the clinical choices you make.

Methods of Clinical Reasoning

In 1994, researchers Fleming and Mattingly compiled studies creating a cornerstone of research for our discipline, showing that occupational therapists fluidly move between multiple types of thinking while practicing.[10] The data demonstrated that therapists employ different kinds of clinical reasoning to inform specific decisions for specific situations. In the researchers' words, OT decision making "involves creating therapeutic experiences in which patients must deal with very imperfect bodies…and still find some reason to struggle for a meaningful life."[10]

As this quote implies, occupational therapists do not simply treat the cognitive or biological pathology of a condition but instead focus on the condition's impact on the person's life and his or her individual performance goals. For this reason, treatment techniques are seldom the same from client to client, even for clients who share the same diagnosis. So, too, the occupational therapist's clinical decisions must focus beyond producing graded interventions designed to help a client feed himself again—issues of independence, self-concept, and even the social and cultural aspects of eating need to enter into the process.

In general, this "OT brand" of clinical reasoning draws on different methods of reasoning to address different aspects of treating a specific client. It is typical for occupational therapists to switch continually among the different types of reasoning to make decisions and modify interventions throughout the normal course of treatment. As with any skill, most OTs are more comfortable with some types of reasoning than others. But there are times when it is important to be able to use each one to benefit the client. At first, it takes conscious, deliberate thought to use each type of reasoning, but practice helps the process become more automatic and integrated.

The study of clinical reasoning is a worthwhile pursuit in itself, and several well-written texts on the various methods are available to supplement the information in this book. It is beyond the scope of this text to review the theoretical foundations of each reasoning method in detail. Even so, it is important to be familiar with the basic methods and general applications of each so that you can use them effectively as you develop the cases in this book. The rest of this chapter presents a summary of six basic methods of clinical reasoning:

- Procedural reasoning
- Narrative reasoning
- Pragmatic reasoning
- Ethical reasoning
- Interactive reasoning
- Conditional reasoning

Variations occur in both the ways that different texts group the types of reasoning, and the ways they describe them. The primary sources used in the following summary are Fleming and Mattingly's *Clinical reasoning: Forms of inquiry in a therapeutic practice* (1994)[10] and Schell and Schells' *Clinical and professional reasoning in occupational therapy* (2008).[11]

Procedural Reasoning

In practice, procedural reasoning encompasses several areas that may already be familiar to you. In this form of reasoning, decisions are based on an understanding of scientific evidence that gives confidence in an expected outcome. Procedural reasoning is most often used by occupational therapists when making decisions regarding assessment tools and treatment interventions to address an individual's occupational performance problems. Interventions are chosen based on information that reinforces confidence that the intervention will actually help the client. Such decisions should never be based on guesswork—in fact, it would be unethical to decide, "I don't know what to do, so I will just try something." It is essential that treatment choices always be based on sound reasoning.

Just as research includes varying levels of evidence, so procedural reasoning encompasses various types and "levels" of reasoning. The first two types are deductive and inductive reasoning.

Deductive Reasoning

Deductive reasoning takes what is already well known and researched and draws from it logical, reasoned conclusions about what is likely to happen. An example of using deductive reasoning in practice is deciding to use interventions that directly incorporate a well-researched protocol of hand exercises into therapy to improve a client's active range of motion (AROM) after flexor tendon repair. The outcome is directly related to the decision to use a specific protocol, and results should be fairly predictable. Likewise, deciding to provide dementia patients with a calming room when they are agitated based on conclusive evidence in multiple studies demonstrates the use of deductive reasoning.

Occupational therapy training acquaints students with many well-researched assessments and interventions for standard conditions. But what if there are no well-researched occupational therapy interventions for a condition? What if the tools in the treatment setting are not standardized? What if the client has a goal for treatment that you are not familiar with? Any of these variations may indicate that it is time to turn from deductive reasoning with its well-researched findings toward inductive reasoning instead.

Inductive Reasoning

Inductive reasoning projects a less certain outcome than does deductive reasoning, because the result is implied or generalized from one or more indicators that a *similar* approach was effective in treatment. For this reason, it might be considered a lower "level" of reasoning. Using the previous hand surgery again as an example, if the client enjoys video games and the activity analysis indicates that the hand motion used during the games would increase the client's AROM in a manner similar to that in a well-researched exercise protocol, it would be reasonable to conclude that having the client play video games as part of his therapy will lead to the desired results. No protocol or research exists that documents the efficacy of playing video games for therapy after this particular hand surgery, but the positive outcomes could be inferred from related research and task analysis of the movements needed to play the video game. Because of the creative nature of occupational therapy and the need to customize interventions to each client's unique context, inductive reasoning may be an appropriate choice more often than deductive.

As with levels of evidence, the lowest level of procedural reasoning with the weakest rationale is a clinical decision based on personal experience or someone else's clinical experience alone. If no published evidence is available to show that this treatment works, there is a lower confidence level that it will result in a positive outcome for the client. However, when no other evidence is available, clinical decisions made on the basis of personal experience or that of others can still be considered "knowledge-based," even though the risk of not getting the desired results is increased.[11] This is one reason why occupational therapy and occupational therapy assistant programs as well as the AOTA place a heavy emphasis on developing evidence and promoting the use of evidence-based practice,[12] so that therapists can more often use procedural reasoning with higher confidence levels due to the availability of solid research to support our clinical decisions.

With all types of procedural reasoning, it is important to keep your knowledge up to date through the use of evidence-based practice. New evidence is published continually to help therapists improve their treatment based on higher levels of scientific evidence. However, this research can help clients only if the occupational therapist takes responsibility for finding and assessing it seriously.

It might seem as if clinical reasoning should stop here, with procedural reasoning. However, the definition of evidence-based practice is based on three things:

- the published evidence of an intervention's effectiveness,
- the practitioner's clinical expertise, and
- the client's values.[13]

Considering this, procedural reasoning alone is not enough to ensure effective evidence-based treatment that is *client-centered*. Knowing how to treat a condition through the use of procedural reasoning does not provide enough information to understand anything more about the client than simply his or her symptoms and diagnosis. The five methods of clinical reasoning presented next provide a more dimensional understanding of clients and their conditions.

Narrative Reasoning

The foundation for providing client-centered intervention is truly knowing the client. If an intervention is to be customized to the client's unique life in all its contexts, the therapist must know about that unique life in detail. Narrative reasoning is the process used to help the therapist understand what the client is experiencing and how it is affecting his or her daily life.[11] In Fleming and Mattingly's[10] early 1994 study, narrative reasoning was found to be one of the main types of clinical reasoning to influence occupational therapists' thinking.

The narrative process helps clients express who they are and make sense of what is happening to them. By listening to them and demonstrating that what they are sharing matters, the therapist validates who they are. Engaging clients in the narrative process is also one of the most effective ways to establish a collaborative relationship with clients, a vital part of working with them toward a newly imagined future.

The first challenge in using narrative reasoning is determining how best to engage the client in sharing his or her perception of what is happening. Even if the client's physician has provided a thorough report about the client's health issues, it is still critical that the therapist hear what is happening from the client's perspective. It may be helpful to start by saying something like, "I see from the information the doctor sent that you have a fractured wrist. There's an x-ray report here too, but I'd like to hear about what's going on from you, since you're the one it's affecting. Can you start by telling me what happened?" After carefully listening to what the patient says (and noting what he or she *doesn't* say), a good follow-up might be, "Can you tell me how this has affected you and your normal routines?"

This storytelling process that results from such questions not only encourages the client to describe the illness experience from his or her own perspective but also provides a glimpse into how the client is responding emotionally to the health challenge, what the client feels are the most important activities that have been interrupted, and what the client thinks future life might be like. Be cautious when a client says something that does not sound correct—remember, the client's interpretation is personal and subjective. For example, if a client says, "I don't think I'll ever get better," it is unwise to contradict or to try to change the client's mind, even in the interest of offering hope. What is important is the feeling that has been expressed, the emotional truth he or she feels right now. It is far better to validate what a client has said and appreciate their distress than to tell them they are wrong to feel that way. The opposite may also occur, as when a client after a catastrophic accident expresses a goal that is likely to be unrealistic—for instance, when a man who has suffered a high-level spinal cord injury states, "I'm determined to go back to work as a construction worker." On hearing this, the therapist might validate the client by saying, "It sounds like you really enjoyed your job, and that you are very determined to get better. Tell me what you liked most about it?" Through ongoing narrative during the treatment process, the client may come to modify his goals as he redefines who he is and what a meaningful future life would be like.

What if someone is unable to share a personal narrative verbally? Perhaps the individual has an intellectual disability, is so depressed he or she is unable to carry on a conversation, or has a breathing tube impairing verbal communication. Narrative reasoning is still possible in such circumstances and may be especially effective if the person wants to communicate but has been unable to do so. The narrative process will require creativity on the therapist's part to help the person express him- or herself nonverbally. The person might be able to write about what he or she is experiencing or draw a picture of it. The therapist might need to interpret nonverbal body language offered in response to questions. Some interesting articles have been published about using music, dance, and theater to help people narrate their experiences.[14]

With procedural reasoning, it is fairly easy to decide what to do with published information or expert opinions that speak to the effectiveness of certain interventions—such information guides the choice of interventions used. But what does a therapist do with the information from a client's personal narrative? What kinds of clinical decisions can this information be used to inform? The case study in the accompanying box will help you explore answers to these questions. As you read Angela's story, attune yourself to what she is expressing about her life. When you have finished reading, make a list of the following:

- Indications of what Angela's life was like before the accident
- How Angela feels about her current medical condition
- Activities and relationships that are important to Angela
- Angela's occupational performance goals for the future

CASE
1.1

CLIENT:	Angela, 21-year-old female
CONDITION:	Thoracic level four spinal cord injury (T4 SCI)
SETTING:	Inpatient rehabilitation facility

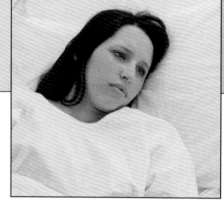

Angela is a 21-year-old female patient who has been admitted to an inpatient rehabilitation facility following a complete thoracic level four spinal cord injury (T4 SCI) as a result of a motor vehicle accident. She was a passenger in the car her boyfriend was driving when the accident occurred, and she was the only one hurt. In therapy, she expresses the following to you:

> I actually don't remember what happened. There must have been a problem with the car, or else someone else did something stupid, because my boyfriend is a really good driver. I don't know why he hasn't been in to see me yet. He's probably going to dump me now because he thinks I'm a freak in a wheelchair. God, I can't even go to the bathroom by myself anymore! My parents hate him–they think he did this to me. But I really, really want to talk to him. If we could just talk, maybe we could still make it work.
>
> I feel like a prisoner here at the rehabilitation center. I don't know why I couldn't just go home when I got out of the hospital. My parents can take care of me until I can get back to college. I'll have to share a bedroom with my sister again–that will be horrible, we fight constantly. My roommate at college is probably wearing all of my clothes. And look at me in this ugly hospital gown. Maybe it's better that my boyfriend doesn't see me like this.
>
> I'm studying to be a research physicist. My parents are both scientists, so being a "brainiac" runs in the family. I've got a 4.0 GPA going. Now I'll probably have to drop out. My life is like a disaster! I might as well just call it quits if I have to live the rest of my life like this. All my friends are at school. Everything seems so hopeless.

What questions would you ask Angela after reading her story? Narrative reasoning is used to help you decide how to probe further and encourage clients to think more deeply about different areas of their lives. It is also used throughout your client interactions to create further dialog that will allow clients to continue expressing their changing understanding of what is happening to them as treatment progresses. Through the narrative process, you will help clients revise their unique personal stories and project future goals and expectations. This vision of a future self is critical to inspiring the client and helping him or her remain invested in doing the difficult work to reach that imagined future life.

When listening to clients express their personal narratives, it is important not to judge what they say as "right" or "wrong," "good" or "bad." In the words of Schell and Schell, "The client's story is like a compass that indicates a direction in which to begin intervention."[11] The narrative is a starting point from which the therapist can help the client move forward. Using the earlier example of Angela, consider questions such as these:

- How would you get Angela to discuss her feelings and values?
- Would what you heard guide your priorities in making treatment decisions?
- Which activities of daily living (ADLs) do you think would be most important to Angela?
- How might you involve significant individuals in Angela's therapy?
- How would Angela's long-term occupational performance goals guide this phase of her therapy?

In narrative reasoning, therapists use reflective listening (clarifying what the client or patient seems to be trying to express) while supporting and encouraging the client to consider the outcomes of therapy and to develop a life story of a meaningful future based on them. What might a realistic future life story be for Angela? The interventions a therapist designs for his or her clients reflect as much narrative reasoning as procedural reasoning.

Pragmatic Reasoning

Pragmatic reasoning consists of the practical, mundane, real-world decisions involved in arranging for and delivering therapy to clients, such as scheduling therapy sessions and deciding on the best way to use the tools available in a particular treatment setting to meet clients' needs. These decisions represent the creativity, compromises, and adjustments the therapist makes throughout the workday to juggle busy schedules, work within budgets, and meet bureaucratic requirements while still looking out for clients' best interests. Some aspects of pragmatic reasoning are as follows:

- The immediate work environment presents some of the most obvious pragmatic decisions. This includes the physical work space in which treatment is provided, the personnel available within the setting, and the conditions such as policies under which service is conducted. Personnel include other disciplines on the interprofessional team, and the skills of the other rehabilitation staff who are available. For example, if one of the rehabilitation staff is certified in wound treatment or sensory integration, he or she might provide guidance that would lead the therapist to adjust interventions on a particular case.
- Pragmatic decisions will also be based on the equipment available, the amount of time allotted for treatment, and the productivity requirements the therapist must meet. The availability of a treatment kitchen or bathroom for working with clients on ADLs might have a positive impact on the therapist's ability to prepare clients to return home independently. If such facilities are not available, then pragmatic reasoning is needed to adjust interventions for the client. Will the bathroom on the residential unit serve instead? Or would it work to bring a commode chair into a private area of the gym for practice?
- Pragmatic clinical decisions are also influenced by the broader healthcare environment in which the therapist is treating. This environment includes insurance coverage for different types of occupational therapy services, copay amounts, and state and federal healthcare policies. Any of these can and will influence the treatment provided. For example, if a client runs out of paid therapy visits or cannot afford copayments, the therapist may suddenly need to design a home program or train a friend of the client to be a therapy partner. If a treatment is available that would

benefit a client but insurance will not pay for it, therapist and client are faced with a clinical decision. Pragmatic reasoning is used to make these types of decisions. To new therapists, some of the constraints of the practice context may seem nonnegotiable and restrictive. However, a creative approach to sharing equipment and space, coordinating care, and compromise can lead to solutions that will improve clients' outcomes even in challenging circumstances.

- Pragmatic decisions also include those based on the therapist's understanding of the unique skills, abilities, preferences, and attitudes—both positive and negative—that he or she brings to the therapeutic relationship. Treatment decisions that are based either wholly or in part on the therapist's own needs are not necessarily wrong or bad. Sometimes they are simply practical or necessary. For instance, the therapist must consider treatment decisions that have a personal impact, such as travel distance or the need to include time to eat. For therapists practicing in a home care setting or traveling between multiple school or clinic settings, logistics such as the timing of a lunch stop have to be considered even though they may affect treatment. If the therapist can provide treatment in a particular setting at only a certain time of day and this presents a problem for the client, then pragmatic reasoning is needed to help decide how best to proceed. If a client would benefit from a certain skill in which the therapist is not well versed, should the client be transferred to another therapist who does have the skill? Sometimes, that is the simplest solution, whereas other times extenuating circumstances prevent it. If that is the case, what then? Is it possible to consult with a therapist who has the necessary skill, or can the skill be learned or strengthened?

- Self-awareness about one's own preferences and attitudes is also an important part of pragmatic reasoning. For example, a therapist who is unaware of his or her own attitudes about clients and their needs and goals, or who does not recognize his or her own needs and goals, can unwittingly influence treatment negatively. Self-awareness comes from personal reflection and an ability to be open and honest with oneself when faced with feedback from others.

Self-awareness and the Johari Window

The Johari window[15] is a self-awareness tool developed by two American psychologists to help people better understand themselves and improve interpersonal relationships. This technique uses a four-paned window to represent the personality. One pane contains traits that both we and others know about our personality. A second pane contains personality traits of which only we are aware. A third pane holds traits we *don't* know about ourselves but of which others are aware and could tell us. The fourth pane holds traits that are completely unknown to both ourselves and others.

In an occupational therapy context, this technique speaks to the therapist's need for self-honesty, the need for self-awareness about how the attitudes and biases *we know about in ourselves* affect our clients, and the importance of asking others for feedback about what they observe in us *that we might not be aware of.* At the same time, it is important to maintain an open and vigilant self-observation about how our own attitudes and behaviors affect the treatment decisions we make. One way to do this is to periodically ask oneself, "Why did I make that choice? Is it truly in the client's best interest, or do I want to do it that way because it is most comfortable for me?" Once we recognize our own biases and the negative impact they can have on treatment, we can be proactive and make decisions to prevent that from happening.

A personal story will illustrate. I was raised in a fairly conservative family in which physical privacy was strictly observed. Although I had both a brother and father in my home while growing up, I had a real lack of practical knowledge about the male body, and my science classes went only so far. In being honest with myself as an occupational therapy student, I discovered that I was completely unnerved by the thought of working with a male client on personal care skills. As luck would have it, my second fieldwork placement was at a Veterans Administration (VA) hospital. I knew that if I wanted to succeed in my role, I had to deal with my fears about doing ADLs with male clients. Before I left for my fieldwork placement, I met with my college OT advisor and told her about my misgivings. She did not dismiss my concern as trivial or say that it would work itself out with experience. Instead, she suggested that I visualize doing an actual personal care treatment that I had learned in class with a male client, and we would talk about what I anticipated would be the most uncomfortable aspects. Then we problem-solved practical ways to get through it: how to focus, and what to say and do in different scenarios. When I arrived at my fieldwork site, I approached my clinical supervisor with a plan. I acknowledged my inhibitions, shared the work I had done in preparation, and asked if I could initially be assigned clients who needed personal care as part of their treatment but who might not be fully aware of my nervousness. She agreed, and after successfully treating several difficult dementia clients, I had the confidence and skill I needed, and my supervisor complimented my problem-solving skills and self-awareness.

Even after many years of experience, therapists can and should continue to learn and grow in self-awareness about personal biases. Asking oneself questions such as those that follow, and answering them honestly can be an effective way to explore one's own attitudes.

- How would I feel if I treated someone who had been imprisoned for hurting another person? Or a brain-injured client whose drunk driving caused her own accident?
- Do I have prejudices or biases about certain cultures or personal characteristics? People on public assistance? People who are morbidly obese? If so, what are my feelings, where do they come from, and how might they affect the way I deliver care?
- How do my political, cultural, and religious affiliations influence my attitudes? How might they affect my therapeutic relationships with clients and their treatment outcomes?

And, most importantly:

- What can I do to make sure my values and opinions do not harm my clients? Whom can I talk to, what can I read, are there other sources to help me with this?

Ethical Reasoning

It is a curious thing that some clinical reasoning texts do not include a discussion of ethical reasoning. This omission may reflect not an oversight but an assumption that being ethical in one's reasoning is so much a part of who the occupational therapist is and what he or she does that it literally goes without saying. In fact, the Occupational Therapy Code of Ethics is intended specifically as a "guideline for ethical decision making."[16] It is included here as a separate method of clinical reasoning to ensure that students consciously consider the ethical aspects of their clinical decisions. Some ethical decisions are difficult and may be stressful for both therapist and client. Advance preparation in sound ethical reasoning skills can help ease the difficulty.

When considering ethical decisions as a type of clinical reasoning, it is important to take into account the context of treatment and the types of ethical decisions that are likely to emerge. In some settings, committees, boards, or individuals are responsible for assisting with difficult ethical decisions. Such committees will routinely handle conflicts related to medical ethics, end-of-life decisions, and breaches of clients' rights. If such a group or individual is available, they may be of assistance in the event of a difficult ethical issue. However, there will be times when smaller or more immediate ethical decisions emerge in the midst of treatment, and skills are needed in the moment to deal effectively with these decisions. The following discussion explores some common ethical decisions that arise in practice—issues related to confidentiality, autonomy, justice, veracity, and fidelity.

Confidentiality

The following is a true story about confidentiality that has been altered to protect those involved:

> A therapist we will call Jodi goes home, and her father asks her if their neighbor is still in the hospital because he wants to stop in to see him. Without thinking, Jodi says that the neighbor has just been discharged. After the father stops in to see the neighbor, the neighbor mentions the visit to his daughter Anne. Anne is not happy that her father's discharge was discussed outside the hospital, and she complains to the hospital administrator, telling him that Jodi did not protect her father's right to confidentiality. When interviewed, Jodi is honest and admits to the slip. She is fired from her position for a HIPAA violation, even though she has worked for the facility for many years and has a spotless record.

The choice of what information to share demonstrates both the therapist's ethical reasoning and ethical standards.

Occupational therapy students are dismissed from fieldwork placements; employees are disciplined, denied promotions, or fired; and therapeutic relationships are destroyed through inadvertent slips of the tongue. In a healthcare environment, staff members must be hypervigilant about protecting all clients' rights to privacy. Decisions about whom to share information with should be made on a need-to-know basis—and for the occupational therapist, this means following certain guidelines:

- Discuss a client's information only with employees on that client's interprofessional team or those who are involved in another professional capacity with this client. Billing personnel may need to know certain types of information about the client, but not other information.
- If a consultation with another therapist is needed to discuss an aspect of patient care, stick to the topic, and do not discuss unrelated patient information with the other therapist.
- Do not leave patient charts or patient information on a computer screen where others can see them.
- Do not talk about patient information in elevators, hallways, cafeterias, or other areas where others can overhear.
- Do not discuss client information with the client's family or friends unless the client has given permission to do so.
- Consider in advance what you will say if a client sees someone they know in the treatment room and asks about them.

- Protect yourself by not asking for any information unless you have a direct professional need to know it. When you see someone you know in the elevator at work, it may be natural to say, "Hi, what are you here for?" but train yourself not to ask.

Protecting yourself also means you cannot look up information on whether your neighbor had her baby yet, or the results of your grandmother's test. Most hospitals monitor online access to patients' records, and it is possible to determine who viewed what records at which times. Don't take the chance—the price you may pay is not worth it.

Maintaining privacy in small towns can be extra challenging, especially if the therapist lives in that town. People may get upset if you don't share information—they may think asking about neighbors is being considerate, not nosy. Get in the habit of cutting people off mid-sentence before they can even say a name. Make a joke out of it by saying, "I can neither confirm nor deny whatever it was you were going to ask," and leave it at that. If they persist, tell them, "I don't want to get fired, so please don't ask me anything about my job." That blunt approach—sometimes even with family members—usually works well.

These are just a few examples of the kinds of ethical decisions that arise almost daily. As a therapist, you must find you own ways to guard against slips and protect yourself and your clients.

Autonomy

Autonomy is the right of individuals to make decisions about their care and their lives, and it extends to making decisions that others might consider bad, unhealthy, or unsafe. Such decisions could include clients' desire to return home even though they are unable to care for themselves independently, the choice to refuse treatment that evidence indicates would benefit them, or the right to make life choices such as smoking that will worsen their condition. Therapists may face an ethical decision when the responsibility to do no harm (nonmaleficence) is in direct conflict with a client's freedom of choice.

The right to refuse treatment, including therapy, is one that all therapists will certainly encounter. If you work in a skilled nursing facility or a mental health or other residential facility, it may be part of your role to go to clients' rooms and take them to therapy. What do you do when a client says, "No, I don't want to go to therapy?" The client has a right to refuse, so do you just walk away? Do you trick the client and say, "We're going to the dining room, not to therapy?" What is the best way to respect the client's rights while at the same time respecting his or her right to choose?

To resolve this dilemma, the first step is to make sure the client's decision is an informed one. In cases of impaired cognition, the client's right to independent choice remains intact if he or she can understand on a basic level the consequences of that choice. If a client's ability to understand is in question, there may be an agent or health-care guardian who has the right to choose on the client's behalf. If the client is not adequately informed, some education may need to be provided about the possible benefits of treatment and the consequences of refusing it. The second step is to understand why the client is making this choice. With the client who refuses to leave his room to go to therapy, is he afraid he will be too far from the bathroom? Is he afraid therapy will hurt? Is he concerned that he will miss a visitor? Or does he have an underlying mental disorder such as depression or paranoia that keeps him from wanting to leave his room? Listening carefully and asking questions to help clarify the client's perspective may create an opportunity to address these concerns. Perhaps therapy could be provided in another area or at another time. Ultimately, after every reasonable attempt has been made to understand the client's perspective and encourage him to attend therapy, your decision must respect his ultimate right to autonomy.

The therapist is never required to provide any treatment that he or she deems unsafe—in fact, it would be unethical to do so, even if the client desires it. When acting in accordance with a client's wishes poses a risk of harm to the client, then guidance from the clinical supervisor or ethics committee may be necessary. In some cases, such as when a client wants to be discharged home and the healthcare providers deem the discharge unsafe, there may be policies and procedures in place to cover it, such as specific documentation stating that the discharge was made "against medical advice." Such policies are generally followed to provide some level of protection from liability for the facility if the client's health suffers as a result of the decision. Sound ethical reasoning will lead you to investigate and follow such safeguards.

Justice

The ethical principle of justice in health care generally refers to providing care in a way that is fair to everyone who receives treatment. This includes decisions that allow equal access to services, such as avoiding discrimination in the way clients are scheduled or in decisions about which staff member works with which clients. For example, it would be unjust and unethical if clients of low socioeconomic status were always scheduled to see therapy assistants after the initial evaluation, whereas clients of higher socioeconomic status were always scheduled to see licensed therapists. Ethical reasoning might also come into play when deciding what to do when a client does not call to cancel an appointment or routinely arrives late for appointments, thus affecting other clients. What is the ethical decision to make in such a case?

Veracity and Fidelity

Veracity and fidelity are the ethical principles that guide the therapist's truthfulness, honesty, and commitment in providing service. It might seem that being honest with a client is a given, but some of the most difficult ethical challenges a therapist can face involve just such decisions. For example, what if a family member says, "Dad doesn't know he has cancer (or is terminal, or is not going home), and we don't want you to tell him." Suddenly you are in the midst of an ethical dilemma—how can you be honest with your client and also honor the family's request? Or what if a client asks, as soon as the two of you are alone, "Am I going to die? I can't get anyone to be honest with me!" In both cases, ethical reasoning tells you that the client has a right to be treated with honesty.

Such problems usually can be addressed with diplomacy, honesty, and negotiation. Asking questions rather than giving answers is usually an effective approach. For instance, with the family members you might ask, "Do you think your dad already has a pretty good idea about his health?" or with the client who wants to know whether he or she is terminal, ask, "What do you think? Tell me about it."

Ultimately, responsibility may need to be put back on the care coordinator, such as the physician or the family. In such cases, you might tell the client something like this: "It sounds to me as if you have a lot of reasonable questions. I think you should have a good discussion with your doctor (or family) and be up front." Then, tell the client that you are going to give the physician or family a heads-up that he or she already has a clear sense of the issues and is going to be talking to them. Encourage everyone to be honest. Family and sometimes even medical practitioners are concerned that if clients know that their diagnosis is terminal or that an undesired change is about to occur in their health or living situation, they will give up. The family or physician may need support themselves to understand that clients may make decisions about the time they have left that are different from what others might wish, and that even if the client does "give up," that also is their right.

Two additional aspects of veracity and fidelity are being honest with clients about expected recovery and keeping promises made to them. Be cautious not to "overpromise" in an effort to make a client feel better in the moment. If evidence indicates that a client will likely have residual deficits after recovery, ethical reasoning dictates that you must be honest with the client about that. You can still assure the client that you will work hard to help him or her improve as much as possible, and that you will keep working to figure out how to help him or her cope with any remaining deficits. You may frame your response by stating that recovery is always an individual process and is never completely predictable, but that a typical recovery for the condition would be "X." Ethical reasoning may turn out to be the one method of clinical reasoning that keeps you awake at night.

Interactive Reasoning

Some excellent books have been written about the importance and process of interactive reasoning.[7] At its core, interactive reasoning reflects choices the therapist makes with regard to initiating, fostering, and supporting an ongoing therapeutic relationship with each individual client. How should the therapist approach a new client and start the relationship? How would a client describe the therapist's "bedside manner?" Even though certain aspects of individual personality are set to an extent, therapists can still employ different approaches and techniques with a client when doing so would be beneficial. Developing this kind of versatility with interactive reasoning requires practice.

For the therapist, another important aspect of interactive reasoning involves realizing that every client will need different things from the client–therapist relationship. A smile and gentle touch may be all one client needs to continue working hard in therapy. Another client will need boisterous and frequent approval, while yet another may need limit setting and even confrontation to help them succeed. Active listening, an important concept typically included in occupational therapy training programs, is one of the skills involved in interactive reasoning. Other interactive skills include trust building, affirmation and validation, genuineness, confrontation, and empathy. To decide which skills to use, therapists must be able to attune to and connect with clients, in order to understand what they are feeling and what they need. As noted earlier in this chapter, the importance of establishing this connection is supported by the OTPF-III, which recommends that the therapist develop an intentional relationship with each client through therapeutic use of self, empathy, and client-centered collaboration.[2]

Developing a collaborative client–therapist relationship is an effective way to support the client in achieving his or her goals. Fleming and Mattingly[10] describe the important role a collaborative practice style plays in gaining a high level of commitment from the client. Employing such a style often means that the therapist shifts the therapy process from "doing to" the client initially, to "doing with" the client, to finally having the client "do for" him- or herself. Even when working at the bedside of an unresponsive client, the therapist can develop a relationship of teamwork and collaboration. Using the pronoun "we" instead of "I" (e.g., "Next, we're going to work on getting your joints moving."), explaining the treatment and the reasons for it to the client, and including some of the client's preferences (discovered perhaps through a chart review or conversation with the family) are ways to communicate respect and empathy and foster an atmosphere of collaboration.

True teamwork implies that control and power are shared. When a client has been traumatized and has been admitted to a healthcare setting instead of going home, the therapist and the facility hold virtually all the control and power. It is up to the therapist to make clinical decisions that will help "level the playing field of power and control." Giving the client choices is one important way to do this. Another is to make sure that goals, plans, and interventions are meaningful and significant to the client. Both of these are ways the therapist can use interactive reasoning to empower and motivate clients to engage in therapy.

Conditional Reasoning

In describing conditional reasoning, Schell and Schell[11] state that therapists "must flexibly modify interventions in response to changing conditions." Another way to describe this kind of reasoning is to call it "thinking on your feet"—being flexible while therapy is happening in order to make adjustments during the process so that each treatment is the best experience possible for the client. Of all the reasoning methods discussed here, conditional reasoning requires perhaps the most confidence and experience to do well. After all, therapists put a lot of effort into planning and preparing for treatment sessions. Unless something catastrophic happens, why change the plan? Conditional reasoning challenges the tendency to stick to the "status quo."

Some therapists are committed to carrying out a plan "no matter what," whereas others are naturally more comfortable with an organic flow and a flexible plan. Regardless of the therapist's personal comfort zone, the skillful use of conditional reasoning can offer clients tremendous benefit. What if the client did not sleep well last night and has low energy? What if a treatment space or piece of equipment is not available? The smart therapist will plan ahead for different conditions, especially with a relatively new client, or one with a condition that varies from day to day. Being prepared with a range of equipment and plans demonstrates strong conditional reasoning, for such preparation makes it possible to grade interventions to be slightly more or slightly less challenging than anticipated for the session. This kind of flexibility and planning is particularly important when customizing the challenge to the client. The treatment session may be only a half-hour long, so being flexible, having a variety of tools at hand, and being prepared with alternative interventions will help to ensure that the client gets the most out of each session.

According to Fleming and Mattingly,[10] the therapist's ability to design interventions to meet multiple goals is also an aspect of conditional reasoning. An example will illustrate this important skill.

Mary is a 28-year-old woman who suffers from recurrent, severe depression. At the short-term mental health inpatient facility where she is hospitalized, Mary receives occupational therapy as part of her treatment. It takes a great deal of encouragement to get her to come to the OT room and engage in any activities. Mary's short-term occupational performance goals are aimed at increasing her ability to express herself verbally, taking the initiative to perform self-care tasks, and increasing her attention span during occupational tasks.

Stanley, Mary's occupational therapist, has been going to her room in the morning and working with her on bathing and dressing, and then trying to get her to attend OT in the afternoon to work on her other two goals. Mary still needs a lot of prompting and is often passive during dressing and hygiene activities. Stanley is also frustrated that he has been largely unsuccessful in getting her to participate in the afternoon small-group sessions, despite his efforts to involve her in groups that are working on plant care, crafts, and cooking, which are listed as interests of hers. He has noticed that Mary seems slightly more engaged during their morning one-on-one sessions than at other times of day, so he decides to leverage her engagement at that time to get her to work on multiple goals with the same intervention.

The next morning, Stanley goes to Mary's room earlier than usual with a basket of her clean clothes that he retrieved from the facility's laundry. He explains that he would like her to help him fold her laundry first and then choose what she wants to wear for the day. Although Mary still needs prompting, she actually asks questions about what he wants her to do. As they work together, she points out that some of the clothes are wrinkled and that she doesn't want to wear them for that reason. Stanley offers to bring an iron the next day so she can iron her clothes, and she agrees.

After the laundry is folded and put away, Stanley prompts Mary to start getting dressed. He tells her he has to leave but that she should finish dressing herself so that she can go to breakfast soon.

Later in the day, Stanley checks in with nursing and learns that Mary did come to breakfast fully dressed. Stanley felt that Mary had made solid progress on all three of her performance goals. Stanley's ability to use a single intervention, engaging Mary with her own laundry tasks to address multiple goals, demonstrated excellent conditional reasoning.

Neuromuscular and orthopedic rehabilitation is another area in which it is especially critical for the therapist to integrate goals related to multiple client factors into the interventions chosen, because doing so imitates the complex interplay of skills the client will need when performing tasks in his or her natural environment. The motor performance skills a client will need to move around and manipulate objects in his or her environment may begin as individual actions that the therapist needs to cue and that the client needs to focus on one at a time. A skilled therapist can artfully select and combine these individual actions with process skills such as initiating, sequencing, and terminating tasks, thus enabling the client to develop effective performance patterns and ultimately achieve his or her desired occupational performance goals.

Clinical Reasoning in Practice

The preceding discussion of "nimble thinking" is a good segue into a closing observation about the applications of clinical reasoning in occupational therapy practice. Fleming and Mattingly's[10] early seminal studies revealed that most practitioners move easily and seamlessly from one style of thinking to another, and that each individual treatment decision may reflect the therapist's use of a combination of reasoning types— for example, a decision the therapist originally reached through pragmatic reasoning also could easily have ethical implications.

As you work with the practice cases in Part II of this text, you will be asked to reflect on a specific case and consider which type of clinical reasoning might serve you well in planning treatment. At times you may find it difficult to use only one reasoning method, and that is realistic. As long as you understand the differences among the various methods and combine them thoughtfully, using more than one type of reasoning can be a practical and realistic way to select the interventions and approach that are best suited to help the client reach his or her goals.

REFERENCES

1. Schell BAB. Professional reasoning in practice. In: Gillen G, Scaffa ME, Schell BAB, eds. *Willard and Spackman's Occupational Therapy*. 12th ed. Philadelphia, PA: Lippincott Williams & Wilkins; 2014:384.
2. American Occupational Therapy Association. Occupational therapy practice framework: domain and process (3rd ed.). *Am J Occup Ther*. 2014;68:S1–S48. http://dx.doi.org/10.5014/ajot.2014.682006.
3. Taylor RR, Van Puymbroeck L. Therapeutic use of self: applying the intentional relationship model in group therapy. In: O'Brien JC, Solomon JW, eds. *Occupational Analysis and Group Process*. St. Louis, MO: Elsevier; 2013:36–52.
4. Kielhofner G. *Conceptual Foundations of Occupational Therapy Practice*. Philadelphia, PA: F.A. Davis Company; 2009:8–14, 65–83.
5. National Board for Certification in Occupational Therapy. A practice analysis study of entry-level occupational therapist registered and certified occupational therapy assistant practice. *Occup Ther J Res*. 2004;24:S1–S31.
6. Sladyk K, Jacobs K, MacRae N. *Occupational Therapy Essentials for Clinical Competence*. Thorofare, NJ: Slack.; 2010:80–81.
7. Schultz-Krohn W, McHugh Pendleton H. Application of Occupational Therapy Practice Framework to Physical Dysfunction. In: Schultz-Krohn W, McHugh Pendleton H, eds. *Occupational Therapy: Practice Skills for Physical Dysfunction*. St. Louis, MO: Elsevier; 2013:40.
8. Schkade JK, Schultz S. Occupational adaptation: toward a holistic approach to contemporary practice, part I. *Am J Occup Ther*. 1992;46:829–837.
9. Law M, Baptiste S, McColl MA, et al. The Canadian Occupational Performance Measure: an outcome measure for occupational therapy. *Can J Occup Ther*. 1990;57(2):82–87.
10. Fleming MH, Mattingly C. *Clinical Reasoning: Forms of Inquiry in a Therapeutic Practice*. Philadelphia, PA: F.A. Davis; 1994.
11. Schell BAB, Schell JW. *Clinical and Professional Reasoning in Occupational Therapy*. Philadelphia, PA: Lippincott Williams & Wilkins; 2008.
12. Lin SH, Murphy SL, Robinson, JC. Facilitating evidence-based practice: process, strategies and resources. *Am J Occup Ther*. 2010;64:164–171. http://ajot.aota.org/Article.aspx?articleid=1862647.
13. Sacket DL, Straus SE, Richardson WS, et al. *Evidence-Based Medicine: How to Practice and Teach EBM*. New York, NY: Churchill Livingstone; 2000.
14. Stephenson RC. Promoting self-expression through art therapy. *Generations*. 2006;30:1:22–24.
15. Luft J. Group Process: An Introduction to Group Dynamics. 2nd ed. Palo Alto, CA: National Press Book; 1970.
16. American Occupational Therapy Association. Occupational therapy code of ethics (2015). https://www.aota.org/-/media/Corporate/Files/Practice/Ethics/Code-of-Ethics.pdf.

Case Development Protocol

In practice, you will carry a "caseload" made up of the different clients you will be responsible for treating, with the method for assigning clients to a therapist varying from setting to setting. During the first part of your fieldwork placement, you will likely start with only one or two clients on your caseload, with more added as your training progresses. The thought of treating 6, 10, or even 12 or more clients a day, along with all the related paperwork, can seem overwhelming.

This chapter presents a Case Development Protocol—a multistep process that will help you think through and gain confidence in the practical and professional aspects of evaluating, planning, and delivering treatment to a client from start to finish. The "Case Development Protocol" boxes that appear with the chapter headings summarize the main steps discussed within that section. Each main step is presented as a question. The "Developing Your Case: Step by Step" boxes within the discussion itself break down each main step into substeps. The substeps consist of a list of questions and other guidance to help you develop your case in more detail. A summary of the complete sequence of steps and substeps is included in Appendix B of this text.

The Case Development Protocol is designed to be used as a learning tool to help guide your work with the patient cases presented in later chapters. The accompanying questions will prompt you to analyze your case, make clinical decisions, plan treatment that is client-centered, and provide appropriate documentation. You may be given additional assignments in class to help you develop your skills further by applying the steps quickly across a broad spectrum of conditions or settings. Overall, the Case Development Protocol will help you gain confidence and skill in thinking critically and applying different types of clinical reasoning. The rest of this chapter takes you step by step through the Case Development Protocol process. Let's begin the process by assuming that a new client has been referred to your practice setting and you have been assigned to the case. You have access to the referral form and some background information about the person. How do you begin?

Identifying Relevant Information in the Record

CASE DEVELOPMENT PROTOCOL STEPS 1–6

The six initial steps in developing your case help you consider the kind of information you need by type:

STEP 1	What demographic information do I have for my client?
STEP 2	What information can I find about my client's primary condition?
STEP 3	Does my client have any secondary conditions?
STEP 4	What information can I find to make my client more than just a diagnosis?
STEP 5	Who else will be on the interprofessional team?
STEP 6	What is the preliminary plan for my client after discharge?

Occupational therapists (OTs) use a client-centered, individualized approach to treatment. There is no single "recipe" to follow, even when a treatment protocol is used. The goal is to help clients "get their lives back," or in the case of habilitation, to help clients create the meaningful lives they desire. To accomplish this goal, the OT's treatment must be aimed at working toward specific activities that are meaningful to each client. This cannot be done unless interventions are based on relevant information—information that goes far beyond a simple diagnosis.

How do you get the information you need? Expecting that you will obtain all the necessary information from your client during your first visit is probably not realistic. For one thing, the amount of time you will have for a treatment session may be very limited in some settings. Consider, for example, a referral for a client who has just suffered a head injury and is in the intensive care unit (ICU). You may have only brief periods to work with your client—as little as 5 to 10 minutes, with interruptions for critical care. But undoubtedly you will have access to either an electronic or a paper-based medical record that contains information about the client's condition, status, and overall medical care. Always read whatever background information is available before you see your client. This not only helps you know what condition(s) you should focus on and what questions you want to explore with the client, but also allows you to identify safety precautions and limitations to activity. If the record lists any diagnoses, medications, or symptoms you are not familiar with, you will want to research them *before* seeing the client.

> **Developing Your Case** | **STEP 1**
>
> *What demographic information do I have for my client?*
>
> **1.** Review your case and list the basic demographic information.
> **2.** What other basic information do you need that is not in the case description? What other source(s) might supply this information?

Whether your setting is home care, day treatment, or a school or community center, when you receive a new referral you will usually have access to at least some background information about the individual in advance of your first visit. Although you will not finalize your decisions until you meet with and assess the client in person, being able to carry out preliminary planning and gather evidence-based information are steps that prepare you to be organized, observe appropriate safety precautions, and get the most out of your first visit.

The background information on your client may be extensive, existing as part of a complex electronic record, or may be limited to a few lines on a referral form. Both situations can present challenges. If you have access to large amounts of information, you must be able to identify which information is relevant and which is not. If you are given too little information, you may need to find additional sources to get some of the information. Knowing what kinds of information you need at the outset can save a lot of time. The first six steps in the Case Development Protocol indicates the information you need by type.

Let's think about the potential importance of demographic information. This is often placed at the very beginning or introductory section of a form or record and includes basic identifying information about the person to be treated, such as full name, age, contact information, insurance coverage, as well as perhaps information about your client's race; any ethnic, cultural, or religious affiliation; and next-of-kin. You may need some of this information for insurance or billing purposes as well as for record-keeping, depending on the filing system where you work. Some of this demographic information may also affect your treatment decisions. Take age, for example— how would your approach change if you knew the individual you were treating was 16 years of age, versus 45 or 85 years of age? You might adjust everything from your choice of assessment tool to the types of interventions, to make them appropriate developmentally. Information in this initial demographic section may also give you some ideas about the person's financial circumstances at the time the information was gathered, and any resources available to the person as he or she recovers.

If important information is missing from the documents available to you, then you will need to look for other sources to provide it. These might include:

- direct interview;
- discussion with others on the interprofessional team; or
- discussion (with permission from the client) with other persons of significance such as family and friends.

When accessing any information about clients, take care to use ethical reasoning and respect Health Insurance Portability and Accountability Act (HIPAA)[1] laws! Your clinical supervisor will guide you in following procedures to make sure you protect the individual's rights as you gather information to assist in making treatment choices.

Beyond basic identifying information, perhaps the first thing you think about when you receive a new referral is the condition or diagnosis that you will be expected to treat. Although this sounds straightforward, referrals such as "Wrist pain—evaluate and treat" are not uncommon, and give you little to go on. Such cursory information leaves you with a lot of questions and severely limits any preliminary ideas you may have about what assessments and interventions would be best.

In such cases, you can start by looking at who recommended the therapy and why. Was it a self-referral, or did another professional recommend occupational therapy? This is an important question, because the referral source can make a difference to your approach. For example, if a client self-referred, he or she probably had some reason to believe therapy would be of benefit. If the client expects to receive a certain type of treatment or to experience a particular outcome, it is important for you to know that, and you will want to discuss these matters with the client as you make your initial treatment plans. On the other hand, if a surgeon referred a case to you, you will want to know before you see the client if the surgeon wants you to follow a particular protocol.

Other important aspects of the primary condition to know about may be how long the person has had the condition, how severe it is, and, perhaps most importantly, how it has manifested itself in this particular case. OTs often end up treating the symptoms of the primary condition, and these can vary greatly from client to client. For example, for a client with a fractured wrist, your interventions would not include retrograde massage if the person did not have edema as a symptom. Similarly, for a person with a mental disorder, you would choose different treatments depending on the type or severity of his or her symptoms. Knowing as much as possible about the client's current condition thus can help you with preliminary planning prior to your first treatment session. If this basic information is not available when you receive the referral, you may need to use your pragmatic reasoning to find it. Ask yourself: who might have records on this client's conditions? how would you access them?

If your client's records are extensive, you might find information on the client's condition in the sections on history and physical or medical reports on recent tests or treatments. You might also look to see if other professionals have been asked to assess the individual for the same condition. Although you may not have the training to understand the details of individual tests or exams, the summary reports often provide valuable insight into the client's health status. For clients with chronic conditions who have had a long history of treatment, or those with severe injuries for whom

Developing Your Case | STEP 2

What information can I find about my client's primary condition?

1. Review your case and document the primary condition or diagnosis you will be treating. Include any mention of symptoms, and any objective data about the condition or diagnosis.
2. Is all of the information you found relevant to your occupational therapy treatment? Explain your answer.
3. What type(s) of clinical reasoning did you use to guide your answer to question 2?

the members of a large care team all have provided information, the number of tests and reports can be overwhelming. To organize your search, focus initially only on the condition you have been asked to treat and the information that is most relevant to the type of treatment you are likely to provide. An example would be an operative report. If you will be treating the condition for which the person had the operation, then the type of procedure, any postsurgical restrictions, and comments about expected recovery might all be relevant to your treatment. The individual details of the operation, while interesting, might not offer necessary information for the choices you need to make about your treatment. Give more weight to recent information, and to information that will increase your ability to treat the person safely, such as activity restrictions.

Another important consideration as you review information from a variety of professional sources is each professional's area of expertise and potential overlap among the interprofessional team. There are many areas of performance that may be addressed by more than one discipline—for example, eating for a client whose status is post-cerebrovascular accident (CVA). Dietary, nursing, speech pathology, and occupational therapy all may have an interest in evaluating and providing interventions related to eating. You will need to review these areas closely to coordinate care while avoiding duplication of services. Occupational therapy's role is unique and valuable, and the OT needs to collaborate with many disciplines to make sure the client is getting the best care. As you read your client's background information, stay alert for descriptions of symptoms, occupational performance, and interventions by other disciplines. As a guide for differentiating the role of OT, refer to the AOTAs new value statement[2]:

> Occupational therapy's distinct value is to improve health and quality of life through facilitating participation and engagement in occupations, the meaningful, necessary, and familiar activities of everyday life. Occupational therapy is client-centered, achieves positive outcomes, and is cost-effective.

Although too much information can be a challenge, so can too little. It is not unusual to find yourself in a position where you have less information than you would like before you need to begin a client's treatment. In some outpatient clinics, for example, the therapist is handed a new client's folder when the client arrives for the first appointment. If you find yourself in this situation, think "safety first." Ask yourself: given what you know about the person's condition, what information do you need at a minimum to treat him or her safely? Obtaining this information before you provide treatment should be a priority, and you should make every effort to do so. In some cases, the client himself or herself may be a reliable source of safety information, as when allergies are present. However, information related to contraindications or types of surgical repairs may be beyond the client's knowledge or understanding, in which case you may need to delay providing treatment until you can obtain this information from a knowledgeable source. Perhaps a quick phone call will be all that is needed to obtain vital information before you begin. If you do not believe you have adequate information to proceed safely, speak with your supervisor for guidance.

Step 3 in the Case Development Protocol focuses on secondary conditions. In general, secondary conditions are comorbidities or separate but coexisting conditions. Based on when each condition started and/or the reason for the OT referral, the client will likely have one diagnosis listed as primary. However, you need to be aware of other conditions the client may have because they may affect your treatment choices and the client's recovery. If someone with a broken wrist has diabetes as a comorbidity, this would affect your expectations for the healing timeline and may affect the types of interventions or preparatory activities you choose. For instance, if peripheral neuropathy were one of this individual's symptoms related to the comorbidity of chronic diabetes, you would be cautious when choosing any form of heat to relax tight tendons prior to treatment, since the person's sensation is impaired.

> **Developing Your Case**   STEP 3
>
> *Does my client have any secondary conditions?*
>
> **1.** Review your case and identify any secondary conditions, complications, or comorbidities.
> **2.** Will the client's secondary condition affect your treatment of the primary condition? Explain your answer.

Keep in mind that you must closely follow what is written on the referral, and make sure your interventions are aimed at treating the condition or diagnosis listed there. If you wish to treat a different or additional condition, you should contact the referral source and request that he or she modify the referral. If you do not do this, insurance may deny payment for your services. Even if you think the two conditions are related, there could be difficulties with insurance coverage if the referral is not clear. Talk to your supervisor if you have questions about this.

> **Developing Your Case**   STEP 4
>
> *What information can I find to help expand my awareness of my client as a whole person, more than just a diagnosis?*
>
> **1.** Review your case and identify any information related to personal context.
> **2.** Next to each piece of information note what aspect of the person's life it relates to (e.g., support network, cultural affiliation, education, work status, financial status, and so on).

Next, you will want to look for information about your client that provides personal context. Think of this as a way to help you get inside your client's head and appreciate life from his or her perspective. It is true that most of this information will probably come directly from the client. But can you find hints in the background information that give you some insight? Does the record show what kind of job the person currently holds, or if they are retired or a homemaker? Is there mention of significant people in the individual's life? Can you find anything that relates to your client's religious or cultural beliefs or practices? Are there indications of whether the client lives in a rural setting, or an urban one? When you find information that helps expand your understanding of a person's life, you will have a better sense of where to start in your conversation. For instance, if you know that a male client is a farmer with several dependents still living at home who lists his religious affiliation as Amish, you would expect these aspects of his individual context to influence not only his occupational performance goals for treatment, but also the types of interventions that would be most appropriate, as well as other aspects of treatment.

Because each client will have an interprofessional treatment team, it is important to identify who you will be collaborating with in addition to the client. Not only will you need to share information and coordinate care, some of your important clinical decisions may be based on who is on your client's team. For example, if you were working with a client with assistive mobility devices in a setting where the interprofessional team includes a physical therapist (PT), mobility devices may be an area the PT will focus on. If so, you may be incorporating your client's new skill with a mobility device into his or her normal daily routines, but the PT may fit and train your client on the basics of how to use the device. In contrast, if you are in a setting or working with a client whose team does *not* include a PT, you may do the preliminary fit and training on assistive mobility devices, and then proceed to incorporate it into occupational performance. Adjustments in focus require an understanding on everyone's part about the unique role each discipline plays in that setting. While both the Occupational Therapy Practice Act[3] and the Occupational Practice Framework: Domain and Process, 3rd Edition (OTPF Framework-III)[4] provide guidance, there is still room to broaden or narrow your focus. Again, consider the limited time you may have to work with your client—you will not have the time to "do it all," nor are you necessarily the best person on the team to address all the areas on which you might consider working. OTs provide a unique and valuable service in helping clients regain or develop the ability to participate in meaningful occupations. It is up to us to make sure we define our contribution to the team.

The type of information Step 6 in the process asks you to look for has to do with your client's expected course of care, health outcome, and/or discharge plan. In many

settings, the plan for what happens after a client leaves your care begins at the moment of admission. Usually, an individual or even an entire department or committee will oversee and coordinate the discharge planning process. Case managers or discharge planners may perform this role, or it may be part of the responsibility of someone such as a social worker, nurse, or other professional. With certain types of insurance, the person who admits the individual for treatment may have to state, upon admission, an anticipated length of time the client will need to be treated in that setting before he or she can safely be discharged. You may also hear a specific number of days mentioned in terms of "average length of stay" for a particular diagnosis. Some reimbursement models are designed to pay the care provider for treating someone with a specific condition a set amount of money based on the predetermined average length of stay for that condition.

When reviewing a client's chart for this type of information, you may find that the physician's intervention plan indicates what he or she expects will happen in response to treatment, or how much improvement the client's condition is realistically expected to make during the admission. The medical record may include a specific section for information related to both length of stay and potential discharge plans, such as the level of care or setting the client or patient will need after discharge. As the occupational therapist on the team, you will likely contribute significantly to the development of this plan by presenting information related to the patient's ability to care for him- or herself, and the amount of assistance that may be needed for a safe return home. Having some knowledge of the expected outcomes and potential discharge plans prior to beginning your client's treatment will help both you and the client set appropriate occupational performance goals and prioritize objectives.

Developing the Occupational Profile

CASE DEVELOPMENT PROTOCOL STEPS 7–9

STEP 7	What questions do I ask my client when we first meet?
STEP 8	How do I develop the occupational profile?
STEP 9	How will my client's occupational profile affect treatment?

As occupational therapists, we pride ourselves on providing individualized, client-centered care, the foundation for which is the occupational profile we develop for our clients. As you no doubt will have learned early in your occupational therapy program, the occupational profile includes a summary of your client's occupational history, covering:

- Education
- Important roles and social support systems
- Patterns of daily living, including routines and habits
- A description of the client's "natural" environment(s)
- A summary of the client's interests and values
- Any unique religious, social, or cultural characteristics that influence your client's lived experience

This section focuses on helping you develop your client's occupational profile in more detail.

In Steps 1 and 4 above, you identified important demographic and personal information from the description of your case. In an actual referral, you would find similar information during the process of conducting your medical record or background information review. As you begin working with a new client, it is important that you gain a clear understanding of who he or she is, what your client's life is like, how he or she views the recovery or treatment process, what occupations your client finds most important, and what his or her goals are for the future. It is highly unlikely that even a large amount of written background information will provide you with a complete profile. Your next task, then, is to make some decisions about how you will fill in any gaps in your client's occupational profile.

The questions in Steps 7 and 8 will help you augment the information already provided in the case description and explore new areas that you think are important. When asking interview questions at a first meeting with your client, remember to keep your questions open-ended so that you get as much information as possible. The information you obtain is the key to making sure the care you provide is truly client-centered.

After you have developed the occupational profile, you will need to use clinical reasoning to

---

Developing Your Case   STEP 7

What questions do I ask my client when we first meet?

1. Review the basic demographic and personal context information from Steps 1 and 4. Create a list of interview questions you would like to ask your client to complete the occupational profile.
2. Use the Occupational Therapy Practice Framework-III[3] (OTPF-III) to help you think of other areas you may have overlooked that could be important to your client. Add questions from this review to your list of interview questions.
3. Comment on the techniques you will use during the interview to gain your client's trust and develop a therapeutic relationship. (In other words, how will you employ Therapeutic Use of Self and interactive reasoning?)
4. What type of clinical reasoning influenced you in developing your list of initial interview questions?

Developing Your Case | STEP 8 |

How do I develop the occupational profile?

1. Jot down notes about the client's likely answers to your interview questions from Step 7. Using your interactive reasoning skill, try to appreciate the individual's lived experience, including the illness experience.

2. Using the demographic and other background information from your previous case review as well as your projected answers to the interview questions, develop a 1- to 2-page occupational profile of your client. Make sure to include all relevant areas from the discussion above about what is included in an occupational profile. Refer to this profile throughout the remainder of your case, as it will represent your client.

Developing Your Case | STEP 9 |

How will my client's occupational profile affect treatment?

1. Referring to the profile you developed in Step 8, discuss the implications for occupational therapy treatment by answering this question: "Now that I know the information from my client's occupational profile, what types of modifications will I need to make to my assessments, interventions, or treatment approach?"

decide what to *do* with the information you have obtained. Developing interventions and treatment approaches that are based on your client's unique occupational profile is what makes your treatment "client-centered." Information in the profile can lead you to modify your choice of tools or procedures, your interventions, or your approach. For example, consider how it might inform your treatment to know your client's education level. If your client is highly educated, your clinical reasoning skills might guide you to challenge her to read a scholarly article related to treatment and then discuss it with you. Conversely, if your client has very little education, you might modify home education materials to make them more easily understandable. Or consider a different example involving your knowledge of the client's religious affiliation. If you knew from your record review or interview that a client is an orthodox Jew, sound clinical reasoning and cultural sensitivity would lead you to discuss how you could conform a cooking activity to his or her dietary practices. Or, knowing that a client is angry or shy could also suggest that you should adjust your approach. Time spent developing an occupational profile, either formally or informally, will allow you to customize your interventions and treatment approaches to ensure that your client receives client-centered occupational therapy. In turn, this will lead to increased engagement by your client in therapy.

Preparing for Evidence-Based Practice

CASE DEVELOPMENT PROTOCOL STEP 10

| STEP 10 | How will I prepare for evidence-based practice?

You have already spent a good deal of your academic career learning about a multitude of different health conditions and how to assess and treat them. Yet, even if you have a remarkable memory and a thorough understanding of all the conditions you have studied, someday you will receive a referral to treat a client with a condition you have never heard of. A few years into my first job as an OT, I received a home care referral for a young woman with Werdnig-Hoffmann disease. I had no clue what this was.

Imagine yourself in a similar situation. You might consider handing such a referral off to another OT. But what would happen if you handed off every referral you were uncomfortable with? That would not contribute to your own development, and it certainly would not lead to your being a strong member of the rehabilitation team. The key to successfully treating a condition with which you are not familiar is twofold: research the condition using scholarly sources (such as recent textbooks, journal articles found through internet research, and the like); and use your inductive reasoning skills to consider assessments and interventions for symptoms you have learned about for similar conditions.

In the case of my own referral, I discovered that Werdnig–Hoffmann disease is a rare progressive spinal muscular atrophy disorder with gradually increasing loss of muscle strength and coordination that starts with the extremities but that typically proceeds without cognitive impairment. In school, I had learned about treating amyotrophic lateral sclerosis (ALS) and muscular dystrophy, both of which are progressive neurologic disorders with some of the same symptoms as Werdnig–Hoffman disease. With this knowledge, I worked closely with the client to develop a plan for (1) stabilizing her weak muscles to give her more control of the limited use she had of her upper extremities, head, and neck; and (2) modifying and adapting meaningful activities she wanted to continue doing. These included improved seating and assistive technology to aid in mobility and use of a computer with a mouth stick.

All therapists have conditions we are more comfortable treating, and all therapists will treat clients with conditions we know little about. We have an obligation to give our clients the best service we can. In part, this means ensuring that we have a thorough, up-to-date understanding of the conditions before we begin to treat. Depending on your employer, you may or may not have access to scholarly databases. The American Occupational Therapy Association (AOTA) website (http://www.aota.org) is a rich source of systematic reviews and evidence-based resources to which all members have access.

Developing Your Case | STEP 10

How do I prepare for evidence-based practice?

1. Review academic and other scholarly sources to familiarize yourself with your client's primary condition. Compare the information you find to that supplied in your case to determine which specific symptoms your client displays.
2. Review scholarly sources for up-to-date evidence-based treatment information. Summarize your findings. What do you think about these findings? Are the results generalizable to this setting and this client? How does this information guide you or inform your occupational therapy treatment choices?
3. List preliminary ideas for assessments you might administer to your client.
4. What type(s) of clinical reasoning did you use in creating your list for question 3?
5. What preliminary thoughts do you have about a conceptual practice model that might work well for clients who have this primary condition? Explain.

Projecting the Impact of the Condition on Performance

CASE DEVELOPMENT PROTOCOL STEP 11

STEP 11 What effect will the primary (and secondary) condition(s) have on my client?

In Steps 1 through 10 of the Case Development Protocol, you developed a general understanding of your client's health condition and his or her unique client profile. Now it is time to use your clinical reasoning to apply the information you have gathered and other aspects of care to complete the assessment of your client in preparation for planning interventions.

Even if you are working in a clinic where treatment is based primarily on biomechanical theory, you need to start your assessment by identifying the broader occupational performance goals you are working toward. Since the focus of occupational therapy is to help clients engage in valued occupations, pragmatic reasoning suggests that you begin your goal planning by considering which occupations your client's primary condition has disrupted. You will use both procedural and interactive reasoning to anticipate the likely impact of your client's condition(s) on occupational performance.

Developing Your Case | STEP 11

What effect will the primary and secondary condition(s) have on my client?

1. Using the occupational profile you created in Step 8 and your knowledge of your client's health condition(s) from Steps 2 and 3, describe the impact of the primary and secondary conditions on your client's activities of daily living (ADLs), instrumental activities of daily living (IADLs), work, play, and leisure.
2. Describe the illness experience for your client. What do you anticipate your client's attitude will be concerning his or her condition?
3. Describe the likely impact of the primary and secondary condition(s) on your client's future goals.
4. What type of clinical reasoning did you use to answer questions 2 and 3?

Once you have identified which aspects of your client's occupational performance are negatively impacted, you will know what to assess and treat. Your initial assessments will give you enough information to create goals and an intervention plan, but first you must fully appreciate the client's experience.

While studying different conditions, you will have learned a lot from textbooks and other scholarly sources about symptoms, disease progression, and recovery. Procedural reasoning is reflected when you base your understanding and choices on such evidence. However, this understanding is not complete until you use interactive reasoning. Start by asking yourself the question: "How will my client's health condition affect his or her ability to perform ADLs and IADLs that are meaningful to them?" Then use your knowledge of your client's unique characteristics to answer. Does she want to return to walking her dog or to typing on the computer? Does he want to drive a tractor, balance his checkbook, or both?

Setting as Context

CASE DEVELOPMENT PROTOCOL STEPS 12–14

STEP 12	What will the treatment environment be like?
STEP 13	How long will I be able to treat my client?
STEP 14	What will my role be on the interprofessional team?

You now need to apply pragmatic reasoning to explore the impact of the setting on your delivery of occupational therapy. It is important to understand the impact of setting on your approach to treatment, because it provides another layer of context beyond the information you obtained about your client and his or her condition. The type of setting can affect the amount of time you have to work with the person, the total number of treatment days, the space you have to work in, and the resources available to you.

Step 12 in the Case Development Process invites you to begin by considering the physical space you will be using. In the setting for your case:

- Are you likely to work at the client's bedside?
- Will there likely be a roommate and a shared bath? Are there likely to be privacy or noise issues?
- If you will be in a clinic space, will it likely have mostly gym equipment? Children's tables and chairs? Separate areas for different kinds of treatment or activities?

Developing Your Case | STEP 12

What do you anticipate the treatment environment will be like?

1. Describe in detail the likely physical treatment space for your case.
2. Describe the impact of the physical space on your treatment: what pragmatic decisions will you need to make to use the space you have most effectively?
3. Describe the types of equipment and supplies you will most likely have available to you in this setting.

- What adjustments will you need to make to work in this space, such as coordinating with nursing or other therapists to gain access to the space, or using only equipment that you can carry with you?
- What kinds of equipment will you most likely have available in this setting: common household tools? puzzles and writing tools? gym equipment and other modalities? fine motor and manual crafts?

If you are unfamiliar with the type of setting for your case, how can you find out the information you need to become familiar with it? It is likely that either other students in your class or your OT faculty will have worked in a similar setting—now would be a great time to interview them. Most people enjoy sharing their experiences and knowledge with others.

Step 13 in the process considers available time as a treatment resource. Different settings have significantly different lengths of stay (LOS). In some inpatient settings, you will work with clients whose conditions have an average LOS as short as 2 or 3 days, such as joint replacements. In other settings, such as a day habilitation setting for individuals with cognitive disabilities, the average LOS may be many years.

Treatment time for an individual session can also vary greatly from setting to setting. In an intensive care setting, you may have only 15 minutes at a time with a client, once or twice a day. In many outpatient settings, it is common to have initial evaluations scheduled for 1 hour and subsequent treatments booked in half-hour blocks of time. In day treatment settings where clients remain in the facility for a large portion of the day, or in residential settings such as group homes or nursing facilities, you may have access to clients all day but will plan your occupational therapy treatment for group or individual sessions of a half-hour or 1 hour at an appropriate time.

When treatment time is limited, staff must carefully prioritize how to use the resource of time. This includes carefully choosing the occupational performance goals to be worked on, the assessments and interventions to be used, and the activities the client will do on his or her own. We will address these areas further as we develop the intervention plan.

Many times you must coordinate with other staff strategically to accomplish your goals. Are there nursing rehabilitation aides who can help a client practice new self-care skills between treatment sessions? Can you have an attentive family member get involved? Coordinating and collaborating with other disciplines may also help you manage time. In each instance, you must consider what the *most* important areas for occupational therapy intervention are.

Your role on the interprofessional team is another aspect of the practice environment or setting

---

Developing Your Case | **STEP 13**

How long will I be able to treat my client?

1. Estimate the average length of stay (LOS) for your setting for a person with the same condition as your client.

2. Describe how long your treatment sessions will likely be and how frequently they will occur (e.g., once a week in a 1-hour group session; once a week for a half-hour private session).

3. Using pragmatic reasoning, describe how these time frames will affect your treatments. What adjustments or priorities will you need to make to ensure you use your therapy time with your client as effectively as possible?

Developing Your Case | **STEP 14**

What will my role be on the interprofessional team?

1. In Step 5, you identified the disciplines that will likely be on your client's interprofessional team. Now describe each discipline's major focus with your client, including occupational therapy in the list.

2. What effect, if any, do you think the other disciplines on your client's team will have on your OT focus?

2 Case Development Protocol

that can affect your clinical decisions. In some settings, the physical therapist may address positioning or pressure relief issues, whereas in other settings occupational therapy will evaluate needs in this area. In some settings, the occupational therapist will work with clients to obtain adaptive equipment for the home if it is needed, whereas in some other settings, social workers or other professionals will do this. Being aware of these differences and striving to coordinate care, while making sure you are working within your scope of practice and in a manner that supports occupational performance, can lead to the delivery of efficient and effective care. To achieve this goal, you must be knowledgeable about the interprofessional team in your setting.

Assessment

CASE DEVELOPMENT PROTOCOL STEPS 15 & 16

STEP 15 What specific assessment tools will I use in the evaluation process with this client?

STEP 16 What will the results be from my assessments?

With Case Development Protocol Step 15, it is now time to finalize your selection of assessment tools and methods to use in analyzing your client's baseline performance. Your choices should be shaped by procedural, pragmatic, and possibly even interactive reasoning.

Using your responses from Step 10, review your preliminary ideas about assessments you might administer to your client. Which assessment tools will give you data that will most accurately reflect your client's occupational performance? How much time will it take to administer the different tools you have considered? How well do you think your client will respond to the different assessments based on the occupational profile? Careful consideration of these questions will help you make the best choice.

In addition to the common standardized assessments you will have learned about in class, many others have been created and customized for specific conditions and are available through the Internet at low or no cost. An example is the Spinal Cord Independence Measure[5] (SCIM) for adults with spinal cord injuries (SCIs). The various sections of this tool relate specifically to the performance of individuals with SCIs, making the results more useful in planning interventions for patients with SCI than those of the more general Functional Independence Measure[6] (FIM). Other methods of assessment simply use direct observation of performance as an assessment method—for example, assessing active range of motion for an elderly client with arthritis and dementia by directly observing the client during a dressing activity.

Developing Your Case | STEP 15

What specific assessment tools will I use in the evaluation process with this client?

1. Using the information from Step 10, list each assessment tool or assessment process you want to use in evaluating your client. Next to the name of each tool, identify what the tool is used to measure. Review Steps 10 and 11 to make sure you are including an assessment of all relevant factors that underlie occupational performance, including client factors, performance skills, and performance patterns.

2. Note how much time you think will be needed to administer each assessment, and add up the total time. Compare this time to the amount of time you will have available in one to two treatment sessions. If necessary, prioritize and revise your list.

3. Do your choices of assessment tools fit with the conceptual practice model you suggested using in Step 10? If not, how will you resolve this conflict?

4. List other tools or processes you considered but did not choose. Explain your clinical reasoning for each.

As noted by Trombly, "Occupational therapists are not interested in the exact degree of motion at the hip, knee, or ankle as much as they are interested in whether that motion, for example, allows the individual to transfer to and from a toilet or complete dressing independently and safely."[7]

The downside of using nonstandardized assessments and direct observation, however, is the lack of normative data to compare outcomes to. A sequence of scores for your client obtained over time may be meaningful, but there will be no comparisons to results that would be considered "normal." The lack of normative data for comparison can be a drawback with both insurance companies and physicians if it is not possible to show definitively that the client's performance is outside of what is considered statistically normal. For this reason, many clinics use common standardized tests with all clients in order to obtain at least some normative data.

When choosing the best assessment tools, pragmatic reasoning leads us to look at the time, cost, and ease of administration as additional pertinent considerations. If you do not believe a final score is needed for a normative comparison, you may consider saving time by completing just the parts of an assessment tool that are most relevant. Be sure to employ ethical reasoning by abiding by all copyrights and legal requirements for the tools you choose.

Your initial occupational therapy evaluation typically will take place during the first session or first few sessions with your client. It is a good idea not to fill up the time in the entire first session with assessment activities. If your client has low endurance or difficulty maintaining focus, the outcomes you measure at the end of a session may not be truly representative of your client's ability. In addition, most clients are eager to begin therapy and start making progress, and they may grow frustrated at having to complete a series of assessments. If the assessment results highlight deficit areas, the client might find the results depressing and unmotivating—not a great way to start therapy!

You must also consider that many employers will expect you to formulate a plan of care or intervention plan after your first session with a client. Especially if the setting allows for a longer first visit, you may be expected to complete a basic evaluation form and intervention plan before you leave for the day. Balancing these competing goals requires the use of pragmatic reasoning. First, make sure each assessment you have considered doing is necessary. Is there any redundancy among them? Is there an assessment that will cover several areas? Do you need to perform the entire assessment, or can you get the information you need for the initial intervention plan from just one section of an assessment? Keep in mind that using only part of a standardized form will mean that you cannot use the normative data. For the particular diagnosis or condition, will assessment of underlying client factors along with the occupational profile be sufficient to form the basis of your plan, while other assessments may add depth to your understanding, but could come later?

A final consideration for assessments is how well they "fit" with your client. Knowing your client's occupational profile, how readily will he or she accept the tools you are considering? Will the questions on the assessment tool seem demeaning? Will the vocabulary used in the instructions be too complicated and frustrating? Will the tool require interpersonal, communication, or perceptual skills that are beyond your client's abilities? Use narrative reasoning to determine whether an assessment tool will allow your client to demonstrate or express his or her true abilities, occupational performance goals, and perceptions.

Communicating Assessment Results

Step 16 of the Case Development Protocol asks you to capture the results of your assessments and communicate them clearly. Most clinics have a standard general evaluation form that you will use to document the findings from your evaluations. This form will include information in general categories that are appropriate to the setting: in a physical rehabilitation setting, for example, categories may include functional mobility and self-care, while the form in a mental health setting might include affect, attention span, and interpersonal communication. The general evaluation form will not necessarily include specific scoring data from every assessment tool you used but instead will present it in summary form, while retaining the specific data elsewhere in the client's records. This summary is what other disciplines will read, so your statements in each area must be concise and accurate, reflecting your professional opinion as supported by objective data. Developing Your Case: Step 16 provides specific instructions about how to approach the summary.

For example, you may summarize your findings from a functional ADL assessment by stating on the evaluation form that the client is able to feed herself after setup, needs minimal assistance in bathing and dressing her upper body, and needs maximum assistance with her lower body. Your summary should be supported by your findings from one or more of the assessments you administered. If you are using a scored assessment that would be familiar to other professionals, such as the Functional Independence Measurement (FIM)[6], you can include in your summary the name of the assessment tool and the overall score. In a mental health setting, you would perhaps summarize the person's affect and motivation and refer to a tool such as the Beck Depression Inventory,[8] which would be found in its complete form elsewhere in the record.

You should also consider the need to communicate assessment results to your client. Most clients want to know the results of their tests and what they mean. If the test included a comparative norm, for example, your clients may want to know how they compare. You can and should communicate this information to your client, and using your interactive reasoning skills will help you do so appropriately. Does the client tend to overestimate his or her abilities? Then your delivering performance data in a caring, truthful manner may lead to improved insight and metacognition and help the client set more realistic goals. Does the client lack self-confidence? Then you can use your interactive reasoning skills and Therapeutic Use of Self (TUOS) to determine how you and your client can best work together to improve his or her performance, and to help the client feel good about any progress made.

Developing Your Case | STEP 16

What will the results be from my assessments?

1. Print a copy of the score sheet for each assessment you will use. If it is a nonstandardized observational assessment, create a form to capture your observations. (Tip: Think of the symptoms your client demonstrates, and typical symptoms for this condition.)

2. Review your documentation of the primary condition's symptoms from Step 2, the occupational profile from Step 8, and your description of the impact of the condition on your client's performance from Step 11; then, complete the assessment forms. Use your understanding of the client's condition to make logical assumptions about what results you might see for someone with this condition. Score each standardized form.

3. In paragraph form, briefly summarize your professional findings from the assessments. This brief, professional summary will help the other disciplines on the care team understand the results of your occupational therapy assessment.

Many settings now use electronic documentation, with evaluation forms, plans of care, signatures, and other components all accessed, completed, and filed in a digital format. Often these forms will have predetermined time frames that require you to complete and file the data by a certain date. You may then have an additional period of time to make edits to the form, after which time you will be "locked out." An electronic system usually retains all versions of a form, so take care to use professionalism and integrity in all documentation, even early drafts. If the facility uses only electronic filing, you may need to have paper copies of assessment forms scanned into the electronic record and the paper originals destroyed in an approved manner.

Creating the Intervention Plan

CASE DEVELOPMENT PROTOCOL STEPS 17–22

STEP 17	How do I begin an intervention plan?
STEP 18	What areas should I focus on in treatment?
STEP 19	What are my client's strengths?
STEP 20	What occupational performance goals will my client and I be working toward?
STEP 21	What types of interventions will I use with my client?
STEP 22	How frequently will I treat my client?

The next six steps in the Case Development Protocol focus on the intervention plan and related matters. An intervention plan (sometimes referred to as a treatment plan or plan of care) is designed to provide a concise way to communicate information about OT findings and plans for treatment to the rest of the interprofessional team. The finished document presents a summary of information that generally starts with a list of challenges that interfere with the client's occupational performance and that occupational therapy will address. Some settings will have a standardized form to fill in with this information, others may use an electronic template with dropdown lists to choose from, and still others will require a handwritten paragraph the content of which is determined by a policy stating what to include. Regardless of format, most plans include certain basic elements, such as the client's identifying information, problem areas OT has identified, goals OT plans to address, general interventions to be used in treatment, and the frequency and duration of OT's work with the client.

Policies about the need for a referral vary widely among settings. Some settings do not require a specific occupational therapy referral for a client to receive your services. In this case, your intervention plan will be placed in a location where other members of the interprofessional team can access it. The fact that the client has been accepted into the program automatically grants approval for him or her to access all of the available services. Some settings require the referring practitioner (physician, nurse practitioner, psychiatrist, or other professional) to sign his or her approval and return the intervention plan authorizing treatment before occupational therapy interventions can begin.

In other settings, the referral form itself constitutes authorization as long as it contains sufficient information, and if the OT is providing treatment in accordance with the request, it is acceptable to proceed. The intervention plan still must be sent to the referring practitioner to be signed and returned, however treatment can proceed. In still other settings, payment for treatment can be denied if the OT begins treatment before an insurance agency receives and approves the intervention plan and its supporting documentation. You will need to discuss the specific requirements for this sequence with your supervisor at your particular practice setting.

Developing a List of Occupational Performance Deficits

The list of occupational performance deficits, occupational performance goals, and planned interventions should be created in collaboration with your client. Doing so will increase your client's commitment to the goals and treatment. The client's commitment is essential to long-term success and can be seriously diminished if you simply tell your client what you have decided to do after completing the intervention plan on your own. As with all phases of treatment, this dialogue to establish occupational performance goals and an intervention plan will require your use of interactive reasoning skills and TUOS. You may need to compromise and modify some of the goals you feel would be "ideal" in order to customize the plan to meet your client's goals and preferences. Remember that even the best intervention plan is just a meaningless piece of paper unless the client believes in it and works to make it a reality.

The OTPF-III can also play an important role when you are developing your intervention plan. Using the most current version of the Framework as a tool to broaden your thinking is a good way to make sure your plan leads to holistic practice and avoids focusing too narrowly on just a few client factors. For your work with the cases in this book, you will complete an intervention plan just as you would for a physician and others on the interprofessional team. Appendix D provides an intervention plan template to assist you with this portion of your case development. To facilitate your use of the OTPF-III, Appendix B contains a worksheet based on this framework.

Developing Your Case | STEP 17

How do I begin an intervention plan?

1. Using the OTPF-III[3] worksheet in Appendix D, place checkmarks in the boxes next to the categories that you believe are relevant (R), somewhat relevant (SR), or not relevant (NA) for your case. For each item marked relevant, note in the comment section to the right what the implications are—i.e., how does this occupation, client factor, or performance skill apply to this case? Check as relevant only those areas on which you think OT would focus in this setting.

2. Using the Intervention Plan form in Appendix E and your previous demographic information, fill in your client's identifying information at the top of the form.

Developing an Occupational Therapy "Problem List"

Focusing solely on a client's physical or psychological "problems" does not fulfill the holistic approach that OTs ascribe to. Even so, in many settings, a list of functional problems or performance deficits is often the first part of the intervention plan that you will be required to develop. In practice, using a "top down" or holistic approach to developing an occupational profile likely means starting not with problem areas but with either an informal or guided interview such as the Canadian Occupational

Performance Measure (COPM).[9] This early step helps to reveal the client's current abilities and interests as well as his or her challenges in life. It also provides information about the client's unique personal context, including the illness experience and, ideally, the client's performance goals. This step would be followed logically by assessments administered to identify the client's baseline occupational performance. Only then would the OT develop a "problem list" and intervention plan. Even though this sequence of events would be ideal, the following discussion proceeds in the order in which the intervention plan form is usually completed, with deficit or problem areas identified first.

As you develop the list of your client's occupational performance deficits, make sure it includes only those deficits that you as the occupational therapist plan to address. This is important, because most students want to make a long list that doesn't leave out any important problems. However, the list of performance deficits is not meant to include every challenge the client may face, but only those that OT will be treating. For example, your client's occupational profile may reveal that his finances are unstable and he has limited financial management skills. This is an issue that may *affect* OT treatment, but the question is whether it is an issue that you are going to *treat* directly in response to this referral—that is, are you going to set a goal to help this person improve his financial management skills? Consider a similar situation with different clients. If one aspect of a client's bipolar disorder is poor management of personal finances, then it might be appropriate for you to include this on your list of performance deficits. However, if a client with similar poor financial management skills had been referred for OT treatment for a fractured wrist, it would be much harder to justify including financial management in the

list of performance deficits. In another example, if the individual you are working with has poor short-term memory and she was referred to you for treatment of arthritis, you may take her memory problems into consideration by adjusting your intervention or approach—but are you going to directly *treat* her short-term memory deficit? Are you going to teach her compensatory techniques to help her cope with poor short-term memory? Such pragmatic and procedural considerations are important to include when making clinical decisions.

Developing Your Case | STEP 18

What areas should I focus on in treatment?

1. Review the list of your client's symptoms from Step 10 and their impact on performance from Step 11, and create a bulleted list of your client's deficits in occupational performance. Add the list to the OT Intervention Plan.
2. Review your list and revise as needed to make sure it reflects problems that are:
   - related to the condition for which the client was referred;
   - appropriate for OT to address within the given treatment setting and team;
   - reasonable to address within the expected time frame of treatment; and
   - meaningful to your client.
3. Review the OTPF-III[3] with your client in mind. Does this review give you additional ideas about areas that you should address? Are you using "OT language" in your list? Make any necessary adjustments to your list of performance deficits on the Intervention Plan.

Developing Your Case | STEP 19

What are my client's strengths?

1. Review the occupational profile you created in Step 8. Make a bulleted list of your client's strengths and add them to the Intervention Plan.
2. Review the OTPF-III[3] with your client in mind. Does this review give you additional ideas about areas of strength that you might be able to use in therapy? Are you using "OT language" in your list? Make any necessary adjustments to the Intervention Plan's list of your client's strengths.

A second word of caution: For every challenge or problem included in the occupational therapy list of performance deficits, an occupational performance goal and interventions are needed to address it. Thus, when deciding what to include in your final list of performance deficits, you must also consider the expected amount of time you will have to treat your client. For example, if you anticipate that a client will continue rehabilitation in another setting after discharge, you may decide to leave the treatment of IADLs for the therapist in the next setting and spend your time concentrating on important ADLs during the short time you will work with your client. This does not indicate that the IADLs are less important to the client, only that your time to work with the client is short and the two of you must set priorities.

In acute care settings, it can be a big challenge to find the time to work on the occupations that clients find the most meaningful. Dressing, bathing, and feeding may not be at the top of the client's list, but if going out to eat with friends is important, you can design basic feeding interventions with that goal in mind. While the client's long-range goal may be to become able to feed herself a full meal independently when she goes out with friends, your occupational performance goal for the acute care setting may be for her to feed herself a simple meal with adaptive equipment that she finds acceptable to use in front of others. In another example, perhaps you have a male patient who cares little about hygiene or appearance but who is a very private person. Even though he may tell you his most important long-term goal is to drive his car again, he may agree after some discussion that being able to do his own toileting with no assistance in the short term is also very high on his list.

It is also important to review your list and consider the other disciplines on the interprofessional team and their focus with this client, so that the OT problem list reflects those areas where OT adds the most value. Staying focused on the client's occupational performance will accomplish this—for example, although both physical and occupational therapy could easily address a balance issue, the list of occupational performance deficits could express the "problem" as decreased independence in bathing and dressing due to balance deficits. Occupation-based interventions will then address the balance issue during occupational tasks.

Some care plans will also ask for a list or description of the client's strengths and/or resources, such as a strong social network or a previous history of effective coping skills. This list should include characteristics or strengths that will potentially help clients succeed with overcoming, adapting to, or meeting the occupational challenges included in the list of occupational performance deficits.

Setting Client-Centered Occupational Performance Goals

The occupational therapist has ultimate responsibility for designing intervention plans that include goals, but the goals must reflect *the client's* occupational performance goals. For this reason, goals must be created in collaboration with either the client, or the caregiver, or legal representative (such as a parent or guardian) acting on the client's behalf.[4] Depending on the client's cognitive and communication skills, this collaboration can be accomplished in different ways. Discussing what a client wants to be able to do, along with assessment results that reflect his or her current performance, should allow you and your client together to establish goals that are individualized, meaningful, and measurable.

Some employers prefer that their staff use a specific format when writing goal statements, while other settings leave the choice of format up to the individual. A few common formats are Kettenbach's ABCD format,[10] Gately and Borcherdings' COAST format,[11] and RUMBA by Perinchief,[12]. Some settings expect the OT to write both short-term and long-term goals. Your academic program has probably included training on how to write measurable occupational performance goals, in which case your instructor may recommend that you use a specific approach. If you do not receive specific guidance, the recommendations that follow are sound.

> ### Developing Your Case   STEP 20
>
> *What occupational performance goals will my client and I be working toward?*
>
> **1.** Create three to five long-term occupational performance goals for your client, and add them to your Intervention Plan.
> **2.** For each long-term goal, write one or two short-term goals and add them to your Intervention Plan.

Long-term goals are those you expect the client to reach by the time he or she is discharged from your service, or by the time indicated in the script or referral for length of service. According to Sames in *Documenting Occupational Therapy Practice,*[13] occupational therapy goals can be designed to achieve any of the following outcomes:

- restoration of occupational performance
- habilitation (development of new performance skills)
- maintenance of occupational performance
- modification of contexts or activity demands
- prevention of performance deficits
- health promotion

An example of a long-term restorative goal would be: "By discharge, client will be able to dress herself independently with no more than one prompt." In a community setting, a long-term prevention goal might be: "In 1 month, client will be able to consistently identify and carry out learned strategies to prevent falls while bathing."

Short-term goals are milestones along the way to achieving the long-term occupational performance goal (e.g., "By 1 week, client will be able to don socks and shoes independently in 2 out of 3 attempts.") For each long-term occupational performance goal, there should be 1 to 3 short-term goals. All goals should be time-bound, objective, and measurable, and should clearly state what the person will be able to demonstrate when they have achieved the target outcome.

In settings where a person stays for only a few days, goals may not be divided into short- and long-term categories. In such settings, the intervention plan will reflect the occupational performance goals that are expected by the time of discharge, and daily short-term objectives will be incorporated into the daily notes included in the record. In settings where interaction with a client may last for a year or more, goals may be divided up in other ways, such as monthly or by the end of the school year.

Choosing General Interventions

At this point, other members of the interprofessional team who read the OT Intervention Plan will know (1) what you see as the deficits in occupational performance you will work on with your client, (2) your long-term occupational performance goals, and (3) the short-term goals that will help you achieve them. Care plans commonly list the interventions the OT plans to use. In some settings, the referring physician must sign and return the intervention plan before the OT is allowed to treat the client, and he or she limits approval to the OT interventions specified on the plan. In fact, some insurance coverage will pay only for interventions noted on the intervention plan—meaning

Developing Your Case | **STEP 21**

What types of interventions will I use with my client?

1. List on your Intervention Plan the general types of interventions you plan to use. Include passive and active interventions, preparatory activities, and patient education activities.
2. Do your choices of interventions fit with the conceptual practice model you suggested using in Step 10? If not, how will you resolve this conflict? Explain.

that for any interventions used but not included on the list when the plan was created, an amended intervention plan may need to be filed in order to receive payment.

Of course the list of interventions cannot be expected to include every conceivable intervention an OT might employ, but rather the category or general type of intervention, with enough specificity that the reader will have a good understanding of the plan. Terms used on the interventions list should go beyond broad generalities such as *client education*, *therapeutic activities*, and *ADLs* and include the purpose of the intervention along with the type. This will help to ensure the plan's clarity. The following examples are general categories that allow plenty of flexibility, while still communicating a clear purpose:

- Community mobility activities
- Writing activities for dominant hand
- Stress reduction activities
- Energy conservation techniques
- Social skills development group activities
- Home management skills

On the intervention plan, the word *graded* need not precede the name of the intervention, because it is expected that interventions will be graded as the person progresses.

Developing Your Case | **STEP 22**

How frequently will I treat my client?

1. Complete the frequency and estimated length of treatment portion of your Intervention Plan.
2. Sign and initial your Intervention Plan with your professional initials.

Finishing the Intervention Plan

Protocol Step 22 provides guidance on how to finish the intervention plan by addressing frequency of treatment. Your signature is then added to the plan, along with any appropriate professional credentials (e.g., OTS, COTA, OTR/L, OTD) after your name.

If there is a referral form, your plan for the client's frequency and duration of treatment should correspond with the referring practitioner's request. For example, a physician might request that a client be seen twice per week for 1 month. If no frequency or period of treatment is recommended, there may be Medicare or other insurance guidelines or regulations to take into account. Medicare allows a treatment plan to extend as long as 6 weeks if the need is properly documented, whereas an insurance plan may have a cap on the total number of treatments they will pay for in 1 year, with treatments by all therapy disciplines included in that number. In such cases, if your plan was to see a client who is recovering from a CVA 3 days per week for 1 month, and the client is seeing a physical and speech therapist concurrently, an insurance cap may be exceeded in just a few weeks regardless of the length of your projected treatment. In some states, a script is automatically limited to 4 weeks unless a longer period of time is specified on the script. A client's willingness to pay privately for care not covered under insurance is also an important consideration. Such situations can be confusing under any circumstances. While you are still a student, however, it is especially important that you make sure your intervention plan recommends the frequency and time period you believe would provide the most benefit to the client, and then check with your supervisor to determine whether any other parameters may influence the decision.

Insurance aside, it is important to consider how often and how long a client would typically be seen for therapy. Again, this varies by diagnosis and by setting. Generally, the more acute the client, the more frequently he or she would be seen. In some acute settings, the client may be engaged in one or more OT sessions daily, 5 to 7 days per week. A setting that provides intensive rehabilitation might schedule twice-daily sessions of occupational therapy totaling 1.5 hours of treatment time per day for clients who can tolerate it. In other outpatient or residential settings, clients might be seen on a weekly, twice-monthly, or even a monthly schedule.

The duration of a client's treatment also varies by diagnosis and setting. Sometimes, clients who attend day programs for intellectual, psychological, or chronic physical dysfunction continue treatment for many years. Intervention plans to maintain and enhance engagement in meaningful occupations may be effective for several months or longer before they need to be modified. On the other extreme, clients in short-term-stay settings may have intervention plans with occupational performance goals that are intended to be achieved in only a few days.

Frequency and duration may be expressed at the end of an intervention plan as, "OT treatment sessions 30 minutes per day for 1 week," or, in a mental health inpatient setting, as, "Client will attend two OT groups each day for 1 month." The types or purpose of the groups would be listed as the interventions.

Planning the First Five Treatment Sessions

Prioritizing and Managing Time

CASE DEVELOPMENT PROTOCOL STEP 23

STEP 23 | How will my first five treatment sessions be organized?

At this point, the Case Development Protocol calls for putting your assessment and treatment ideas into action. In Steps 15 and 16, you decided what assessments to use and "projected" their outcomes, and in Step 21 you chose the general types of interventions that would meet your client's needs. In Step 22, you determined how much time you had to work with your client in each session. What do you do next? Will you have time to perform all the assessments on the first day you see your client? What specific intervention(s) should you do for the first treatment session? We will demonstrate this process by showing you through the planning of your first five treatment sessions using the case example of Angela from Chapter 1. Then complete the 5-Day Treatment Session Planning Template from Appendix E for your case.

There are several important aspects to planning the initial treatment sessions. First, the assessment results should reflect your client's baseline performance as accurately as possible. Keep in mind the related caveats mentioned earlier in this chapter: the potential effect of the client's acuity and stamina levels on his or her ability to complete your assessments; the client's possible frustration at having to wait to begin the

How will my first five treatment sessions be organized?

1. At the top of each column on the 5-Day Treatment Session Planning Template in Appendix D, fill in the estimated treatment time you will have on each date of service for the setting in your case.

2. Enter the name of the assessment(s) you plan to administer on the first day of treatment. Add the approximate amount of time it will take you to administer next to each.

3. Add assessment(s) to the Plan section at the bottom of the first day, to show what you will do on the second day of treatment.

4. Continue adding assessments as needed for the remaining days. Include any reassessments that are likely to take place in the first 5 days of treatment.

5. Add specific interventions to the first day of the 5-Day Treatment Session Planning Template.

6. In the Plan section at the bottom, make suggestions for what you will work on the next day.

7. Continue filling in interventions for the remaining days.

8. Review your plan. Are all occupational performance goals from the Intervention Plan addressed in the first 5 days? What adjustments would improve your plan? In your case development report, comment on changes or improvements you decided to make to your first draft of the 5-Day Treatment Session Planning Template.

9. What guided you in making these improvements? What type(s) of clinical reasoning did you use?

interventions rather than starting them right away; and the expectation in many settings that you will create the intervention plan after the first or second visit. A balance of all these competing interests is needed, with your first OT sessions dedicated to the most essential assessments, and consideration given to starting some basic interventions with the client, even on the first visit, so long as insurance allows this.

As the sessions progress, you will probably want to administer some additional assessments to enhance not only your understanding of your client's occupational performance but also his or her preferences and occupational performance goals. You will want to repeat assessments periodically to document progress and outcomes. Thought also needs to be given to a "home program" or to work that your client will do outside of treatment sessions. Another important consideration is whether the assessments and the order in which you administer them reflect your conceptual practice model. Starting with a COPM[8] before you perform manual muscle testing, for example, would reflect a "top down," or holistic, approach that evaluates the client's performance and priorities first before assessing underlying deficits.

To illustrate how to plan treatment sessions let's consider the case study of Angela from Chapter 1: the 21-year-old woman who suffered a complete fourth thoracic level (T4) spinal cord injury in a motor vehicle accident. Assume that you are the occupational therapist who received the referral to treat Angela in an inpatient rehabilitation unit. After familiarizing yourself with her medical background and introducing yourself to her, you might consider using the following assessment tools:

1. A COPM[9] to develop an occupational profile
2. Manual muscle testing of upper extremities and trunk
3. An Interest Checklist[14]
4. A modified Functional Reach Test[15] for sitting balance
5. Semmes Weinstein Monofilament Sensory test[16] of upper extremity and trunk, to measure sensory ability
6. SCIM[5] assessment of basic ADLs
7. An IADL assessment including meal prep, laundry, and light housekeeping skills
8. Beck Depression Inventory[8]
9. Community Integration Questionnaire[17]
10. Jebsen Taylor Hand Function Test,[18] to assess grasp and coordination

All of these tests would be relevant to use with Angela, but which should be done first? Should all of them even be used? The first 4 days could easily be devoted to conducting all of these tests, but as discussed earlier, that might not be the best strategy. One possibility would be to prioritize by considering the setting and the other members of the interprofessional team. In this case, assume that the team includes a rehabilitation nurse, a psychologist, and a physical therapist, in addition to the neurologist with whom you will be coordinating care. It is also safe to assume that when you review Angela's chart you will have access to the information from an American Spinal Injury Association (ASIA)[19] classification assessment. The ASIA test indicates Angela's muscle strength and sensory function at a point in time after the spinal cord injury. For a T4 complete spinal cord injury it is likely that the ASIA scale would indicate that Angela has full motor and sensory function of both upper extremities, impaired sensory and motor function in the chest and trunk, and no function or sensation in her lower extremities.

As to the interprofessional team's roles and division of tasks:

- Physical therapy will likely focus on sitting balance, muscle strength in the trunk and upper extremities, and transfers and functional mobility using a wheelchair.
- The psychologist will likely focus on psychological adjustment and coping skills postinjury, as well as any mood disorders such as depression, stress, or anxiety.
- The nurse will monitor Angela's overall health status and work with her on gaining independence in attending to her own health needs, such as maintaining skin integrity, managing bowel and bladder function, and being aware of health risks such as pneumonia, urinary tract infections, and autonomic dysreflexia.
- Occupational therapy's major contribution is in fostering Angela's independence in ADLs, IADLs, and leisure and work occupations.

With this information in mind, look again at the list of assessments.

You will certainly support the work of other disciplines with Angela and even incorporate new learning from their work into your own occupation-based activities. That said, given the minimal time you have available for OT, you can consider letting others on the team take the lead on the depression assessment and even the sitting balance and transfers. Therefore, for now, the Modified Functional Reach Test[15] and Beck Depression Scale[8] can be crossed off your initial OT assessment list. Interviewing your client using an occupational profile will allow you to better understand Angela's goals related to occupational performance, her perception of her current performance level, and her interests and priorities. Since this information can be used to guide the rest of your planning process, the COPM[9] would be a good choice to do first.

Since Angela has just left an acute care hospital to start intensive rehabilitation, she may have barely started to work on independence in basic ADLs. For that reason, it would make sense to start with a baseline of ADL performance and consider delaying both the IADL Assessment and the Community Integration Questionnaire[17] until after Angela has achieved some success in basic ADLs and gets closer to discharge. Based on the ASIA[19] scale, there is no indication that Angela has deficits in her hand coordination or upper extremity sensation, so the Jebsen–Taylor Hand FunctionTest[18] and Semmes Weinstein Monofilament Tests[16] can also be eliminated. The ASIA[19] test would also indicate normal muscle strength in both upper extremities; however, Angela will likely benefit from additional upper extremity strength to help compensate for the loss of her lower extremity function. Although physical therapy will certainly focus on general strengthening of Angela's trunk and upper extremities, you as the occupational therapist will want to capitalize on this strength by incorporating activities that challenge upper extremity strength in your activities. Your activity analysis will also require you to know Angela's baseline strength so that you can adapt activities appropriately. Therefore, it makes sense to perform a manual muscle test of both upper extremities, to gain a better understanding of what Angela can do and how much strengthening or compensation may be necessary as you move forward.

Another review of your initial list of assessments reveals that the SCIM[5] and Interest Checklist[14] remain. The SCIM[5] will assess basic ADL performance, your main focus, so this test should also be one of your initial assessments. The Interest Checklist[14] will give you a better understanding of what occupations will motivate Angela, although this information can also be identified through the COPM[9] tool's leisure and social sections.

The pragmatic clinical reasoning demonstrated above, then, suggests the following sequence and time allotments:

1. Start Angela's assessment by completing a COPM[9]—20 to 40 minutes.
2. Next, move on to a manual muscle test and grip strength testing of both upper extremities—20 to 30 minutes.
3. Administer and score the SCIM[5] after the manual muscle test—30 to 45 minutes.
4. If time permits after the COPM[9], and/or if that test yields insufficient information about Angela's leisure interests, the Interest Checklist[14] may be done. If time is short, perhaps Angela could complete it on her own and bring it back to therapy to discuss it with you.

According to the time allotments above, an estimated 1 hour and a half will be needed to conduct the first three initial assessments. If you don't know from personal experience how much time is needed to administer an assessment, you can usually find the information by doing an Internet search for common standardized tests.

In an inpatient rehabilitation setting such as Angela's, an occupational therapist may have up to 1.5 hours of OT treatment in a day, although the time would most likely be divided between two sessions. Even adding some basic interventions into each of the first sessions, it is clear that within the first 2 days of beginning treatment with Angela, you will be able to complete the first three initial assessments above and also create the intervention plan. You can give the Interest Checklist to Angela later in the week to complete on her own, as is reflected in Figure 2.1, which presents a portion of Angela's 5-Day Treatment Session Planning form. The Interest Checklist appears under Day 4, and a reassessment has also been added under Day 5.

Now, assume that the assessment results from Angela's tests have been used to formulate the intervention plan shown in Figure 2.2. This plan provides the information needed to finish planning the remainder of Angela's first 5 days of treatment, with the objective of selecting specific interventions that both conform to the plan and meet Angela's interests. Figure 2.3 shows the same portion of the 5-Day Treatment Session Planning form as in Figure 2.1, but with timeframes, assessments, and interventions added.

When you use the blank template from Appendix E to complete a 5-Day Treatment Session Planning form for one of the case studies in this text, you will refer to your completed Intervention Plan, your projected assessment results, and the sample 5-Day Treatment Session Planning form portions shown here. You will want to check your plan to make sure it reflects assessments and interventions that will address all of your short-term treatment goals for the client. You will also want to make sure your interventions are client-centered and graded to promote improved occupational performance. Use your clinical judgment to make decisions that are realistic and in your client's best interest.

5-DAY TREATMENT SESSION PLANNING FORM

Patient Name: _Angela X._

Day 1 _1.5 hours total_	Day 2 _1.5 hours total_	Day 3 _1.5 hours total_	Day 4 _1.5 hours total_	Day 5 _1.5 hours total_
Assessments: _COPM_[8] _.5 hr_ _MMT BUE and_ _dynamometer .5 hr_ _Start SCIM .5 hr_	**Assessments:** _Finish SCIM .5 hr_	**Assessments:**	**Assessments:** _Give Interest Checklist_ _to complete on own._	**Assessments:**
Interventions:	**Interventions:**	**Interventions:**	**Interventions:**	**Interventions:**
Plan: _Finish initial_ _assessments._	**Plan:** _Create intervention_ _plan._	**Plan:**	**Plan:**	**Plan:** _Reassess MMT,_ _dynamometer, and_ _SCIM._[4]
HP:	**HP:**	**HP:**	**HP:**	**HP:**

FIGURE 2.1   5-Day Treatment Session Planning Template—Assessments. Note in the highlighted rows that the three initial assessments for client Angela have been completed and preliminary notes on the plan have been added. Day 5's "Plan" block shows that Angela will be reassessed at that point.

INTERVENTION PLAN

Patient Name: *Angela X.*

OVERVIEW: *Angela is 21 years old and was admitted to the inpatient rehabilitation facility on 01/01/2015 after suffering a complete T4 spinal cord injury on 12/10/2014 due to a motor vehicle accident.*

OCCUPATIONAL PERFORMANCE DEFICITS

· *Decreased independence in lower body bathing and dressing due to absence of motor and sensory function below spinal level T4*
· *Decreased independence in IADLs such as care of clothing due to decreased functional mobility*
· *Decreased engagement in leisure interests due to decreased functional mobility*

STRENGTHS

· *High level of cognitive ability; enrolled in college*
· *Supportive family and friends*
· *Absence of comorbidities—otherwise healthy*
· *History of engagement in a variety of interests*

OCCUPATIONAL PERFORMANCE GOALS

LTG: *Angela will dress upper and lower body including setup, with the use of adaptive equipment and techniques, by 4 weeks.*

STG: *Angela will complete lower extremity dressing with minimum assistance and the use of adaptive equipment while adhering to safety precautions in 1 week.*

STG: *Angela will use adaptive equipment and techniques to retrieve clothing of choice from closet with minimum assistance in 1 week.*

STG: *Angela will correctly identify three energy-conservation techniques and explain how they will benefit her in 2 days.*

LTG: *Angela will engage in one leisure activity of interest each day by 4 weeks.*

STG: *Angela will create a list of at least eight leisure interests by 1 week.*

STG: *Angela will identify two physical challenges to engaging in her top two leisure interests and brainstorm ways to overcome the challenges or adapt the activity or method of engagement by 2 weeks.*

STG: *Angela will identify two psychological challenges to engaging in her leisure interests, and two ways to cope with these challenges by 2 weeks.*

GENERAL INTERVENTIONS

· *Adaptive bathing/dressing/hygiene training*
· *Incorporation of wheelchair mobility into ADLs and IADLs*
· *Training in energy conservation techniques*
· *Activities to develop coping strategies for reengagement in leisure skills and community re-entry*
· *Occupation-based upper extremity strengthening activities*

FREQUENCY: *Angela will be seen for occupational therapy 2x/day for a total of 1.5 hours, 6 days per week for 4 weeks.*

Signature: _____   **Date:** _____

FIGURE 2.2 Sample Intervention Plan. Assessment results have been used to help formulate an intervention plan for client Angela.

5-DAY TREATMENT SESSION PLANNING TEMPLATE
INPATIENT REHABILITATION FACILITY

Patient Name: _Angela X._

Day 1 _1.5 hours total_	Day 2 _1.5 hours total_	Day 3 _1.5 hours total_	Day 4 _1.5 hours total_	Day 5 _1.5 hours total_
Assessments: _COPM[8]_ .5 hr _MMT BUE and dynamometer_ .5 hr _Start SCIM[4]_ .5 hr	Assessments: _Finish SCIM[4]_ .5 hr	Assessments:	Assessments: _Give Interest Checklist to complete on own._	Assessments:
Interventions: _Demonstrate/ practice w reacher and send with her to try on own._	Interventions: _Explore AE for bathing/incorporate into showering w shower chair._ _Paint toenails of one foot._ _Reinforce pressure relief during session by practicing wc pushups every half hour._	Interventions: _Practice new transfer skill (introduced by PT) to bath bench for strengthening and skill._ _Bathing w AE._ _Explore long-handled dressing equip._	Interventions: _Incorporate new bed mobility skills (introduced by PT) into adapted dressing. Practice hanging up clothes w reacher for UE strength and skill building._	Interventions: _Discuss Interest Checklist. Choose one leisure interest to adapt/explore. Work w nursing and client on AE to assist w toileting skills and skin inspection._
Plan: _Finish initial assessments._ _Work on bathing and hygiene._	Plan: _Create intervention plan._ _Work on tub transfers and dressing._	Plan: _Advance dressing skills. Strengthening through hanging clothes._ _Give Interest Checklist._	Plan: _AE for toileting and skin care._ _Identify a leisure interest and begin task analysis to adapt._	Plan: _Reassess MMT, grip strength, and SCIM.[4]_
HP:	HP:	HP:	HP:	HP:

FIGURE 2.3 5-Day Treatment Session Planning Template—Interventions. Note in the shaded row that specific interventions conforming to Angela's treatment plan and her interests have been added, and that additional details have been added to the Plan section.

2 Case Development Protocol

Planning a Home Program

CASE DEVELOPMENT PROTOCOL STEP 24

STEP 24   What is the best "home program" to support my client's progress?

"Home program" is a somewhat generic term that is used to refer to all activities the therapist recommends that a client engage in outside the scheduled treatment time to support the goals of treatment. Your client may carry out the home program plans in his or her room in a residential or short-term inpatient setting, at home, or even at work. The goals of the home program might include practicing new skills independently or with support, engaging in activities that will continue the progression of restoring the client's abilities, or engaging in reflection and/or planning activities that would enhance and support therapy. In many cases, to gain the most benefit, your client will need to do the interventions planned for therapy much more frequently than therapy sessions alone would allow. Make sure that all home program activities are clearly understood by the client, and that the client demonstrates satisfactory performance of any new skills in therapy before suggesting it for a home program. Other supportive persons in the client's social network can also become involved in the home program, if they have been properly instructed and demonstrate the necessary competence. If the client has any memory deficits, make sure that all instructions are written down. It is helpful to write instructions for home programs on a brightly colored piece of paper, so that the instructions are easy to find and hard to forget. To jog your own memory, you might put a copy of the home program in the client's chart so that you will remember what you asked them to do.

You may be able to increase your client's compliance with your recommended home program by doing the following:

Developing Your Case | **STEP 24**

What "home program" would best support my client's progress?

1. Add your home program plans to the bottom of the 5-Day Treatment Session Planning Template for each day. Make sure to consider how the client's home environment, social supports, and financial resources might affect the home program.
2. Create handouts to give your client to support his or her progress toward occupational performance goals.

- Make sure the client understands the *purpose* of each activity. What will it help him or her be able to do again? Knowing this will increase the client's motivation to stick with it.
- Incorporate the home program into your client's daily routine. If you want the client to do the home program three times a day, try having him or her do it after each meal. If five times a day, add one more time after work (or after the children get home from school) and once more before bed. It will also help if you can find other ways to link the home program activities to activities that are part of the client's regular routine.

- Designate a certain place that is convenient and visible to store the tools needed for the home program. If the tools are out of sight, they are probably also out of mind.
- Although some people dislike charts and checklists, others find such tracking tools helpful with organizing and remembering activities between visits.
- Whenever possible, use occupation-based activities for increased compliance with the home program.

Figure 2.4 shows the 5-Day Treatment Planning form with home program activities added for client Angela.

5-DAY TREATMENT SESSION PLANNING TEMPLATE
INPATIENT REHABILITATION FACILITY

Patient Name: _Angela X._

Day 1	Day 2	Day 3	Day 4	Day 5
1.5 hours total	_1.5 hours total_	_1.5 hours total_	_1.5 hours total_	_1.5 hours total_
Assessments: _COPM³ .5 hr_ _MMT BUE and_ _dynamometer .5 hr_ _Start SCIM⁴ .5 hr_	Assessments: _Finish SCIM⁴ .5 hr_	Assessments:	Assessments: _Give Interest Checklist to complete on own._	Assessments:
Interventions: _Demonstrate/ practice w reacher._	Interventions: _Explore AE for bathing._ _Use in simulated shower activity._ _Paint toenails of one foot._ _Reinforce pressure relief during session by practicing wc pushups every half hour._	Interventions: _Practice new transfer skill (PT) to bath bench for strengthening and skill._ _Bathing w AE._ _Explore long-handled dressing equip._	Interventions: _Incorporate new bed mobility skills (PT) into adapted dressing. Practice hanging up clothes w reacher for UE strength and skill building._	Interventions: _Discuss Interest Checklist._ _Choose one leisure interest to adapt/explore._ _Work w nursing and client on AE to assist w toileting skills and skin inspection._
Plan: _Finish initial assessments._ _Work on bathing and hygiene._	Plan: _Create intervention plan._ _Work on tub transfers and dressing._	Plan: _Advance dressing skills. Strengthening through hanging clothes._ _Give Interest Checklist._	Plan: _AE for toileting and skin care._ _Identify a leisure interest and begin task analysis to adapt._	Plan: _Reassess MMT, grip strength, and SCIM.⁴_
HP: _Explore uses of reacher._ _Choose nail polish & bring tomorrow._	HP: _Do wc push-ups every hour when out of bed._ _Use AE for showering w assist._ _Paint remaining nails._	HP: _Try dressing AE with min assist when getting ready for bed._	HP: _Complete and prioritize Interest Checklist._ _Use AE for dressing/bathing w standby assist._	HP: _Create plan for what is needed to try adapted leisure interest._ _Cont. using AE w assist as needed._

FIGURE 2.4 5-Day Treatment Session Planning Template—Home Program Activities. Note in the highlighted row that activities for Angela's home program have been added.

When working through your own cases, add your own home program activities to the 5-day Treatment Session Planning form. Activities should reflect what you want your client to do outside the time he or she is with you to reinforce new skills, or to promote rehabilitation and engagement in meaningful occupations.

Daily Treatment Documentation

CASE DEVELOPMENT PROTOCOL STEP 25

> **STEP 25** How will I communicate my daily treatment activity?

Many settings require the OT to maintain daily documentation about the treatments provided. This documentation might consist of a tracking form with space for short notations, checkboxes to mark interventions used, space for specific details about the characteristics of the interventions (the duration of each intervention, amount of resistance, positioning, and the like), and notes about how the client responded to interventions. Completed tracking forms may be filed in the client's permanent record or translated into a summary for other professionals to read. Electronic charts may offer short daily note templates for the OT to use, which may be integrated with the billing system. In other settings, the OT may write longhand notes directly in a paper chart or even dictate a note for someone to transcribe for the record. Regardless of their form, notes should be clear, succinct, and accurate to make sure the rest of the healthcare team understands what OT is doing, how the patient responds to OT interventions, what your assessment of your client's progress or condition is, and what your plan is. In this case, more is not necessarily better. A common student error is to include too much in a daily note. The focus should be on client performance, and your assessment of progress.

Developing Your Case | STEP 25

How will I communicate my daily treatment activity?

1. From Appendix E, use the Daily Treatment Note form to prepare one daily note for each of the first 5 days of treatment for your case.

One common format for daily notes is the SOAP[11] format. "SOAP" is an acronym for the order of information in the note: Subjective, Objective, Assessment, and Plan. Whether or not this exact format is used, information reflecting all four of these components should be included in your note. Although this textbook does not aim to teach documentation, a brief review of the key points for each component may be helpful.

- **S:** Subjective information consists of statements from the client that reflect his or her current perceptions of condition, progress, or future expectations. Information in this section can be as brief as one or two relevant quotes from the client—for example, "I used my right hand to eat last night," or "I'm looking forward to being discharged."
- **O:** Objective data include scores or other results from assessments, direct observations from the OT, and descriptions of the interventions performed. Only concrete, observable information belongs in this section, not personal perceptions or interpretations of what a client feels or thinks. For example, "smiling facial expression" and "inattention to directions" are direct observations. "The patient is not motivated" is not.

- **A:** The assessment section is where the OT uses clinical judgment to suggest interpretations of the subjective and objective information already provided. What does the subjective and objective information mean? Is the patient making progress? Procedural reasoning can help determine whether the rehabilitation is progressing as expected by comparing the client's current performance to any protocols or available standards.
- **P:** The "Plan" section indicates how the OT intends to proceed with the patient at the next visit. Figure 2.5 shows a sample daily treatment note that uses the SOAP[11] format to document client Angela's second day of treatment.

When you are working with the case studies later in this text, use the SOAP note or another note format you have learned to document the client's response to activities you have planned for the first five treatment sessions. Your notes should reflect the outcomes and performance that you would expect in response to your assessments and interventions. At key points during the course of treatment, the OT will need to aggregate or summarize the information from daily treatment notes or tracking forms into a progress note. Payers may require a progress note summary at the end of the time period stated in the referral or intervention plan, in order to continue receiving payment for services. Your progress notes should clearly and succinctly communicate the OT process you used with your client to the rest of the interprofessional team.

Creating a Discharge Plan

CASE DEVELOPMENT PROTOCOL STEP 26

> **STEP 26**   What discharge plan does my client need?

As mentioned earlier in this chapter, planning for discharge often starts at admission. However, initial expectations for discharge may change over the course of treatment, either because of health complications, safety considerations, lack of community support or resources, or the client's own wishes.

When the time comes for the interprofessional team to write a discharge plan, there are two primary purposes for doing so. The first is to communicate information to the person or people who will be providing the client's care after discharge. This may be the client or his or her family, an OT at another facility that provides a different level of care, or a non-healthcare worker who will serve in a caregiver or support role for the client after discharge. The information on the discharge plan typically describes the following:

- the amount of assistance the client needs with different aspects of ADLs or IADLs
- progress and ongoing deficits related to occupational performance
- up-to-date standardized measures
- safety issues, such as risks related to deficits in executive function, safety awareness, and the like
- contact information to use in the event there are questions about the information provided

The discharge plan's second purpose is to make referrals to agencies or services that the client may need once he or she leaves the facility.

SAMPLE DAILY TREATMENT NOTE (SOAP Format)

Patient Name: _Angela X._

OVERVIEW: _Angela is 21 years old and admitted to the inpatient rehabilitation facility on 1/1/2015 after suffering a complete T4 spinal cord injury on 12/10/2014 due to a motor vehicle accident._

SUBJECTIVE:

"I like that reacher you gave me yesterday– I can get things myself now." "At least that's something if I can take a shower by myself."

OBJECTIVE:

Patient used adaptive equipment (long-handled shower brush, hand-held shower head) while showering with minimal assistance for doffing lower body clothing. Patient was able to complete wheelchair pushups x3 in anticipation of transferring to bath bench later this week. Patient was able to explain two pressure relief techniques. Patient was able to paint toe-nails of one foot-demonstrated less depressed affect at end of session as evidenced by increased initiation of communication and positive statements at end of session. The Spinal Cord Independence Measure (SCIM)[4] test was completed, resulting in a score of 19. Lowest scores were in bathing and dressing lower body and bowel and bladder management.

ASSESSMENT:

Patient is gaining skill using adaptive equipment, needs minimal assistance for dressing and bathing lower body. Patient demonstrated improved knowledge of pressure relief techniques. Patient is beginning to adjust to change in physical status.

PLAN:

Complete painting toenails of other foot on own. Tomorrow therapy will work on tub transfers and increasing independence in dressing lower body with adaptive equipment.

FIGURE 2.5 Sample Daily Treatment Note in SOAP Format. The form illustrates documentation for client Angela's second day of treatment.

For the purposes of the present discussion, consider again the example case of Angela. Figure 2.6 shows her sample discharge plan.

As you practice with the case studies in this book, you will establish long-term occupational performance goals in your intervention plan that anticipate your client's performance level at the time of discharge. To enrich your clinical skill development, regardless of your client's condition, assume that your client has some residual deficit at the time of discharge, that he or she will have achieved most but not all of the goals you set together, and that he or she will benefit from some level of continued service after discharge. The details in "Developing Your Case: Step 26" will guide you in completing a discharge summary for your case.

Coordinating and Delegating Care

Developing Your Case | **STEP 26**

What discharge plan does my client need?

1. From Appendix E, use the Discharge Planning Template to complete a discharge plan for your client.

2. Describe any challenges you encountered in developing a discharge plan for your client. Did you need to make any assumptions about your client's support system, resources, or personal context?

3. What type(s) of clinical reasoning did you use in developing the discharge plan? Explain.

4. Create any necessary handouts that will help your client after he or she is discharged. This might include contact information that would be needed in the event of problems, or community resources to support ongoing recovery.

5. Make sure your plan takes into account any relevant secondary conditions.

CASE DEVELOPMENT PROTOCOL STEP 27

| **STEP 27** | How can an occupational therapy assistant and an occupational therapist work most effectively to coordinate the OT services for my client?

In many settings, the licensed occupational therapist carries out occupational therapy interventions through a coordinated effort with multiple personnel, including OT assistants, OT students, and/or rehabilitation aides, all working with a client toward achieving his or her occupational performance goals. Settings have policies and job descriptions in place that describe the roles of all the individuals in these various positions. At some point you may need to decide which aspects of care you will handle yourself and which tasks you will delegate and/or supervise through others. New occupational therapists and therapy assistants often are uncomfortable assuming a leadership or supervisory role with others because they themselves are still at entry level, but sometimes it becomes necessary.

Some facilities have well-defined tasks for people with different titles. For example, some rehabilitation settings team up an occupational therapist with an occupational therapy assistant and assign clients to a specific therapy team upon admission. In other settings, the occupational therapists do all evaluations and the occupational therapy assistants do all daily treatments unless the client needs to be reassessed. In some community settings, the therapist may visit only periodically, and service between visits is provided by paraprofessionals.

Your state's OT Practice Act defines the licensure requirements for occupational therapists and OT assistants and specifies which tasks each can and cannot do. If you are not familiar with your state's requirements that dictate things such as the level of supervision required, who can perform assessment activities and certain treatments such as joint mobilization, and the like, then this is a good time to research your state's OT Practice Act.

As a healthcare professional who makes clinical decisions, you must take care to abide by all applicable regulations as well as your facility's policies. In addition to using

SAMPLE DISCHARGE PLAN

Patient Name: _Angela Clark_ **Identification number:** _1234567_

Referring physician: _Dr. Bancroft Simmons_

Date of admission: _01/01/2015_ **Date of planned discharge:** _02/01/2015_

Primary diagnosis: _complete T4 spinal cord injury_

Occupational performance at onset of therapy: _____

Long term occupational performace goals	**Goal status at discharge**
1. LTG: By 4 weeks, Angela will dress upper and lower body including setup, with the use of adaptive equipment and techniques.	Achieved
2. LTG: By 4 weeks, Angela will engage in one leisure activity of interest each day.	Achieved

Comments on goals not achieved: _NA_

Potential safety issues at time of discharge: _Patient is inconsistent in identifying and observing threats to safety in the environment, including water temperature on insensate tissue and fall risks when completing lower body ADLs._

Recommended placement after discharge: _Home with family (parents)._

Recommended referrals after discharge: _Occupational therapy through home care for continued adaptation of IADLs and reinforcement of safety risks in home environment. Driving rehabilitation when appropriate._

Therapist signature: _Susan Student, OTS_ **Date of discharge summary:** _01/01/2015_

FIGURE 2.6 Sample Discharge Plan. The discharge plan shown is for client Angela.

your knowledge of the relevant regulations, you can also use pragmatic reasoning to help you make decisions about delegating and coordinating care activities. You can also apply ethical reasoning when deciding whether an intervention is within not only your discipline's scope of practice but also your own personal competence.

From a budgetary standpoint, it will be necessary for you to work with others in your department to make the most efficient use of resources, particularly human resources. This also means learning to delegate and supervise appropriately so that support staff are utilized in ways that leverage their expertise for the benefit of both clients and staff. When developing an occupational therapy intervention plan and treatment sessions for your cases, review the information related to your state's policies that define licensure requirements, scope of practice, and supervision requirements. Then, consider your plan for your first five treatment sessions from the perspective of needing to delegate some aspects of care to other members of the rehabilitation team.

> **Developing Your Case** | **STEP 27**
>
> *How can an occupational therapy assistant and an occupational therapist work together most effectively to coordinate the OT services for my client?*
>
> **1.** Consider the setting you are working in and your client's condition. Review your first five treatment sessions. Describe which tasks and activities you would have an occupational therapy assistant do, and which you would have an occupational therapist do.
> **2.** Explain your reasoning. Consider conditional, procedural, and ethical reasoning.

Ethics in Practice

CASE DEVELOPMENT PROTOCOL STEP 28

> **STEP 28** | How will I address ethical issues as I provide care?

Chapter 1 of this book has a section that focuses on ethical reasoning. You will end each case analysis by reflecting on potential ethical conflicts or issues that may need to be addressed as you are implementing your intervention plan.

Nearly every decision the OT makes carries with it some ethical implications—for the client, for the practitioner, or for the agency itself. Often these issues arise from conflicts between competing interests, as sometimes happens when healthcare professionals are striving to provide quality care while meeting productivity standards, or to respect a client's right to choose or refuse care. Providing clients with access to services may sometimes conflict with

> **Developing Your Case** | **STEP 28**
>
> *How will I address ethical issues as I provide care?*
>
> **1.** Review the section on ethical reasoning in Chapter 1 of this book, "Informing Your Clinical Choices."
> **2.** Next, review your case and identify any ethical issues you anticipate a possible need to address as you work with your client.
> **3.** Using your interactive reasoning and TUOS skills, describe how you will address any ethical issues you have identified.

their insurance coverage and thus create an ethical dilemma. Weighing the desires of family members against the desires of clients can also give rise to ethical dilemmas. Such conflicts demand that the OT use clinical reasoning, and specifically ethical reasoning, to resolve them. You will find a variety of processes for methodically resolving healthcare issues outlined in the professional literature, and you may already have been introduced to one or more of them during your academic career. In general, these processes apply the concepts discussed in Chapter 1: confidentiality, autonomy, justice, veracity, and fidelity.

REFERENCES

1. U.S. Department of Health & Human Services. Summary of the HIPAA privacy rule. http://www.hhs.gov/ocr/privacy/hipaa/understanding/summary. Accessed December 10, 2014.

2. American Occupational Therapy Association. Articulating the Distinct Value of Occupational Therapy. 2015. https://www.aota.org/Publications-News/AOTANews/2015/distinct-value-of-occupational-therapy.aspx. Accessed September 9, 2015.

3. American Occupational Therapy Association. Definition of OT practice for the AOTA Model Practice Act. *Am J Occup Ther.* 1999;53:6.

4. American Occupational Therapy Association. Occupational therapy practice framework: domain and process, 3rd edition. *Am J Occup Ther.* 2014;68:S1–S48. http://dx.doi.org/10.5014/ajot.2014.682006.

5. Catz A, Itzkovitch M. Spinal cord independence measure: comprehensive ability rating scale for the spinal cord lesion patient. *J Rehabil Res Dev.* 2007;44(1):65–68.

6. Dodds TA, Matrin DP, Stolov WC, et al. A validation of the Functional Independence Measurement and its performance among rehabilitation inpatients. *Arch Phys Med Rehabil.* 1993;74(5):531–536.

7. Radomski MV, Trombly Latham CA, eds. *Occupational Therapy for Physical Dysfunction.* 7th ed. Philadelphia, PA: JB Lippincott Williams & Wilkins; 2014.

8. American Psychiatric Association. *Diagnostic and Statistical Manual of Mental Disorders.* 4th ed. Washington, DC: American Psychiatric Association; 1994.

9. Carswell A, McColl MA, Baptiste S, et al. The Canadian occupational performance measure: a research and clinical literature review. *Can J Occup Ther.* 2004;71:210–222.

10. Kettenbach G. *Writing Patient/Client Notes: Ensuring Accuracy in Documentation.* 4th ed. Philadelphia, PA: F. A. Davis; 2009.

11. Gateley CA, Borcherding S. *Documentation Manual for Occupational Therapy: Writing SOAP Notes.* Thorofare, NJ: Slack; 2012.

12. Perinchief JM. Management of occupational therapy services. In Neistadt ME, Crepeau EB, eds. *Willard and Spackman's Occupational Therapy.* 9th ed. Philadelphia, PA: Lippincott; 1998:772–790.

13. Sames KM. *Documenting Occupational Therapy Practice,* 3rd edition. Upper Saddle River, NJ: Pearson; 2015.

14. Matsutsuyu J. The interest checklist. *Am J Occup Ther.* 1967;11:170–181.

15. Duncan PW, Weiner, DK, Chandler J, et al. Functional reach: a new clinical measure of balance. *J Gerontol.* 1990;45:M192–M195.

16. Weinstein S. Fifty years of somatosensory research: from the Semmes–Weinstein monofilaments to the Weinstein enhanced sensory test. *J Hand Ther.* 1993;6:11–22.

17. Willer B, Ottenbacher KJ, Coad ML. The community integration questionnaire: a comparative examination. *Am J Phys Med Rehabil.* 1994;73:103–111.

18. Jebsen RH, Taylor N, Trieschmann RB, et al. An objective and standardized test of hand function. *Arch Phys Med Rehabil.* 1969;50:311–319.

19. American Spinal Injury Association. *International Standards for Neurological Classification of Spinal Cord Injury: Key Sensory Points.* Atlanta, GA: American Spinal Injury Association; 2011.

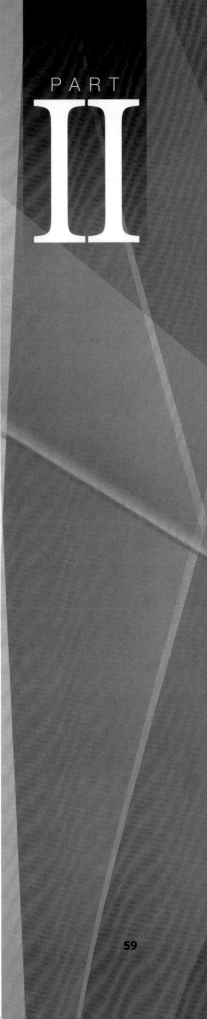

Practice Cases

The cases in Part II are organized in six sections:

- Musculoskeletal cases—including traumatic, repetitive stress, and chronic musculoskeletal conditions
- Neurologic cases—including traumatic, progressive, and congenital conditions
- Cardiopulmonary cases
- Organ system cases
- Mental disorder cases
- Interprofessional cases—demonstrating collaborative skills and coordination of care

The table below provides an overview of all the cases, showing the client's condition as well as the initial practice setting and any other setting to which the client was later transferred to while under the occupational therapist's care. As you practice using the Case Development Protocol with the cases in Part II, you may find that you want to concentrate on a particular condition or a specific practice setting. This table is a useful tool to help you focus your time on areas you most need to target.

Regardless of the setting in which your career as an occupational therapist begins, you will face many of the same challenges as any new employee. But unlike many other careers, occupational therapy relies on your ability to develop a therapeutic relationship with your clients—in fact, it is central to your success in this field. Your ability to use sound clinical reasoning skills builds trust and demonstrates respect for your clients which is important for building the therapeutic relationship. For many occupational therapists, this relationship is also one of the most satisfying parts of the job.

Each case introduces you to the specific setting you are "treating" the client in. You will get to know the client in the same manner that you would in reality—looking through background information, talking with others on the treatment team, and then meeting the client. Each case stops there with a few questions at the end—"Questions as you begin." These represent thoughts or concerns that you might have when you first approach a case. The Case Development Protocol will guide you through developing your case from here forward.

Throughout your career, you will meet many interesting clients and get to know each one in a unique way. The thoughtful use of the cases in Part II will help prepare you to work successfully with them, and will give you the experience to approach your first clients with confidence.

PRACTICE CASES: Clients, Conditions, and Practice Settings

MUSCULOSKELETAL CASES

Traumatic & Repetitive Stress Conditions

CLIENT, CASE	CONDITION	PRACTICE SETTING(S)[a]
3.1 Ivan Petrov	Carpal tunnel syndrome with release	Hospital-based outpatient rehabilitation clinic
3.2 John Cho	Fractured humerus with ORIF	1) Hospital inpatient medical/surgical unit 2) Transfer to skilled nursing facility
3.3 Tyler Babcock	Upper extremity amputation	1) Hospital inpatient orthopedic surgical unit 2) Transfer to outpatient rehabilitation clinic
3.4 Danieka Lawrence	Lateral epicondylitis	Private outpatient rehabilitation clinic
3.5 Yelina Lopez Moreno	Colles fracture with ORIF	Hospital-based outpatient rehabilitation clinic
3.6 Glen Hobart	Flexor tendon repair	1) Hospital inpatient surgical unit 2) Transfer to outpatient rehabilitation clinic
3.7 Thomas Carducci	Total hip replacement	Hospital inpatient orthopedic unit

Chronic Musculoskeletal Conditions

CLIENT, CASE	CONDITION	PRACTICE SETTING(S)[a]
3.8 Sylvia Carter	Rheumatoid arthritis	1) Private outpatient rehabilitation clinic 2) Transfer to homecare service
3.9 Geraldine Johnson	Trigger finger release	Outpatient rehabilitation clinic
3.10 Gerhard Borgman	Dupuytren's contracture	Outpatient rehabilitation clinic
3.11 John Young	Low back pain (herniation between L5 and S1)	Private outpatient rehabilitation clinic

NEUROLOGIC CASES

Traumatic Conditions

CLIENT, CASE	CONDITION	PRACTICE SETTING(S)[a]
4.1 Kendall Murdock	Acquired brain injury	1) Hospital inpatient critical care unit 2) Transfer to inpatient rehabilitation facility
4.2 Richard Kunayak	Left cerebral vascular accident	1) Hospital inpatient medical unit 2) Transfer to transitional care unit
4.3 Janet Lessner	Right cerebrovascular accident	1) Inpatient rehabilitation facility 2) Transfer to homecare service
4.4 Eduardo Rodriguez	Radial nerve injury	Physician-owned outpatient orthopedic rehabilitation clinic
4.5 Miyu Tanaka	Spinal cord injury	1) Inpatient rehabilitation facility 2) Transfer to a for-profit homecare agency

Progressive Conditions

CLIENT, CASE	CONDITION	PRACTICE SETTING(S)[a]
4.6 Sandra Livingstone	Multiple sclerosis	1) Medical model day program 2) Transfer to a skilled nursing facility
4.7 Dale Forsythe	Muscular dystrophy	Homecare agency
4.8 Darnel Parker	Parkinson's disease	Outpatient rehabilitation clinic
4.9 Samuel Duncan	Alzheimer's dementia	1) Medical model day program at a continuing care center 2) Transfer to a skilled nursing facility with dementia unit

PRACTICE CASES: Clients, Conditions, and Practice Settings (continued)

	Congenital Conditions	
CLIENT, CASE	**CONDITION**	**PRACTICE SETTING(S)**[a]
4.10 Theodore Lindstrom	Spina bifida	School-based services
4.11 Sarah Morgan	Down syndrome	Independent contractor serving community residences for cognitively impaired clients

	CARDIOPULMONARY CASES	
CLIENT, CASE	**CONDITION**	**PRACTICE SETTING(S)**[a]
5.1 Elena Gomez	Myocardial infarction with coronary artery bypass graft	Hospital inpatient cardiac unit
5.2 Brandon Greer	AIDS-related pneumonia	1) Hospital inpatient cardiopulmonary unit 2) Transfer to hospice residence
5.3 Boris Schneider	Chronic obstructive pulmonary disease	Homecare agency
5.4 Loretta Thompson	Congestive heart failure	Hospital inpatient cardiopulmonary unit

	ORGAN SYSTEM CASES	
CLIENT, CASE	**CONDITION**	**PRACTICE SETTING(S)**[a]
6.1 Lawrence Timmons	Low vision (open-angle glaucoma)	Outpatient rehabilitation clinic
6.2 Amal Chaudhuri	Burns to hands and face	Hospital inpatient burn unit
6.3 Ronald Knight	Type 1 diabetes with renal failure	Free-standing renal dialysis clinic
6.4 Linda Randall	Cancer with mastectomy and lymphedema	Outpatient rehabilitation clinic

	MENTAL DISORDER CASES	
CLIENT, CASE	**CONDITION**	**PRACTICE SETTING(S)**[a]
7.1 Melissa Clark	Major depressive disorder with suicidal ideation	Hospital inpatient mental health unit
7.2 Roberto Alvarez	Bipolar disorder with manic episode	Mental health day-treatment program
7.3 Erin Batista	Paranoid schizophrenia with psychosis	Home program to support people with chronic mental health issues
7.4 Mary Anne Warren	Posttraumatic stress disorder with alcohol abuse	Inpatient behavioral health program

	INTERPROFESSIONAL CASES	
CLIENT, CASE	**CONDITION**	**PRACTICE SETTING(S)**[a]
8.1 Discharge Coordination Team	Various	Hospital inpatient setting
8.2 Lynnette Wise	Amyotrophic lateral sclerosis	Home hospice program
8.3 New program task force	Homeless outreach service	Grant-funded city agency
8.4 Albert Kirschoff	Diabetes with blindness and above-knee amputation	Outpatient diabetes clinic

[a] 1, Practice setting in which the client first received occupational therapy services.

Musculoskeletal Cases

Traumatic and Repetitive Stress Musculoskeletal Conditions

Treatment of musculoskeletal injuries and syndromes is the "bread and butter" of many medical rehabilitation clinics. These include a variety of overuse conditions, postsurgical treatment for chronic conditions, as well as major and minor traumatic injuries. Only the most serious cases, such as an amputation, will start in an inpatient setting. Even for these more serious conditions, the therapists who work in the inpatient units will often find that they have time for only the most basic treatment before the patient is discharged. In smaller facilities, therapy staff may divide their time between inpatient and outpatient clients. The typical fast pace and variety of both settings are invigorating for many therapists, with a lot of clients demonstrating fast gains in performance leading to relatively short lengths of treatment and high client turnover.

There are also a number of challenges in these settings. The treatment space and equipment are often shared between multiple disciplines, and can be noisy and hectic, with conflicting demands. Although there is frequently a great deal of camaraderie among staff, there is also tension created by the pace and pressure to meet high productivity demands. There can be a temptation in such settings to overbook when volumes are high and staffing is thin. The pace and requirements can also lead rehabilitation staff to be tempted to treat the condition instead of the client, losing the client-centered focus of good therapy. On the plus side, hospitals, medical centers, and hospital-based clinics have the advantage of being able to collaborate with many disciplines, including nurses, social workers, dietitians, and pharmacists, to name a few. In large centers the outpatient clinic may even be located adjacent to offices of the medical practitioners that refer the majority of your clients. This close collaboration can lead to efficiency and continuity of service that benefits everyone.

Most clients in these medical outpatient settings will be referred by primary care and orthopedic medical practitioners. If there is a well-established relationship between the clinic staff and the referring practitioner, scripts (referrals) may be as simple as "Arm pain—evaluate and treat." In other cases, the referral may specify the interventions a practitioner would like to have used with a client, or even a specific treatment protocol he or she wants the therapist to follow. Such specificity should not deter the therapist from using evidence-based treatment, and creative, client-centered interventions. In fact, a difference of ideas on how to approach treatment can lead to valuable communication with the medical practitioner, enhancing the understanding of both parties. Seven different conditions are presented in the cases below, giving a representative sample of some of the most common musculoskeletal challenges you might treat.

CLIENT: Ivan Petrov, 78-year-old Caucasian male

CONDITION: Carpal tunnel syndrome with release

SETTING: Hospital-based outpatient rehabilitation clinic

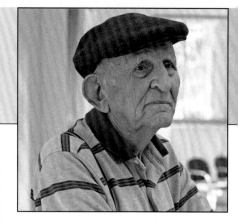

Each morning you receive new referrals to be seen that day in the hospital-based outpatient clinic where you work. The computer printout shows that you will be seeing a 78-year-old Caucasian male with a diagnosis of right carpal tunnel syndrome status post release at two o'clock. The date of the recent surgery is two-and-a-half weeks ago. You also see a note on the intake form from the secretary that the client is a farmer and cannot come to therapy before noon. The referral was made by Dr. Tahir, whom you know well. This particular orthopedic surgeon specializes in hand and arm surgery, and you have treated many of his patients after having an open carpal tunnel release. Dr. Tahir generally does not favor modalities, and encourages patient education and a supervised home program of therapy, along with one to two outpatient therapy visits a week. He usually sees patients in his office again for a follow-up at 6 weeks postsurgery. The referral note also shows that the client has both Medicare Part A and Part B insurance, and his spouse is listed as his emergency contact person. His religious affiliation is listed as Catholic. His home address is listed as a rural route number outside of a small town about 20 miles from the hospital. Ukrainian is listed as Mr. Petrov's primary language, and you notice a hand-written note on the intake form stating that he speaks English, but his accent makes it difficult to understand him at times.

Mr. Petrov arrives early for his appointment, accompanied by his wife, with a soiled, partially intact bandage covering his right hand. He is a large, broad-shouldered man wearing coveralls, a plaid work shirt, and heavy work boots. He appears to be fidgety and uncomfortable in the waiting room. His small wife sits quietly beside him in a faded housedress. You approach Mr. Petrov and introduce yourself, inviting him to accompany you back to the treatment area. He states firmly that he would like his wife Margaret also to come, and you quickly agree, pulling an extra chair into the exam area when you get there.

You begin by asking Mr. Petrov how he normally uses his hands, and how he has been doing since the surgery. Ivan and Margaret, as they ask you to call them, take turns sharing information. The two of them own and operate a midsized dairy farm, along with one of their sons and a hired hand. The son and his wife and their two children live in a house next to the client on the family farm. Although his son handles most of the large equipment now, Ivan still does the majority of the repair work on the machinery, feeds the livestock, and helps with the milking twice a day. His hands had begun to go numb when he was handling tools, and he had noticed increasing weakness and clumsiness. He experienced more pain in his right, dominant hand than in his left, and prior to the surgery, pain in his hands was waking him at night.

Margaret shares with you that she encouraged Ivan to tell his primary care doctor about the problems with his hands when he went in for a bad chest cold a couple of months ago. The doctor suspected carpal tunnel syndrome and referred Ivan to

Dr. Tahir for evaluation of his symptoms. After sending Ivan for a nerve conduction study, they were told that he had mild carpal tunnel syndrome in his left hand, and severe carpal tunnel syndrome in his right hand. After talking it over with his wife, Ivan decided to have the surgery because of his increasing frustration in doing farm work. Now, however, both the Petrovs are wondering if surgery was a good idea because recovery is going much slower than they had expected. When you ask Ivan about the condition of his bandages, he admits that he has been trying to do a little work again so his wife doesn't have to do so much in his place. He explains that even though they use modern, automated milking machines it is still a very labor-intensive process. Margaret admits that at her age it is difficult for her to do a lot of the heavy work, but they can't afford to hire more help. Mrs. Petrov comments that they are both thankful that Mr. Petrov worked at a local factory when they were first married, and so they qualify for Medicare coverage. Even so, the Part B premiums and the copayments are high, and they are concerned about paying for therapy. She tells you the goal of having surgery was for Ivan to be able to continue working on the farm, which is what he loves to do. Ivan mumbles under his breath that he feels "useless" and that he was better off before the surgery.

When asked about how his arm feels now, Ivan tells you his right hand has swelling and tenderness around the incision, and he is still experiencing some numbness and aching at night, although it is not as bad as it was before surgery. He reports that his right hand does not close all the way to make a tight fist, and he has little strength in it. He also says that sometimes when he is trying to use his right hand it shakes. Ivan tells you that weakness and inability to close his fist is his greatest concern, because it limits his ability to repair equipment and work with the milking machines. Other activities he would like to do again are yard work and "getting back to playing my weekly game of poker with the boys!"

Margaret seems embarrassed about the condition of his bandage, and tells you that the doctor said he doesn't have to wear it now, but he isn't supposed to be doing any heavy lifting. Since she knows he's doing more than he should, she says she makes him wear a bandage to keep the dirt out of the healing incision and to provide some protection. Ivan tells you he has some arthritis in his hands, but has never had any broken bones or serious injuries. Margaret reminds him that he has high blood pressure, which is controlled by medication. Ivan reports that he takes Tylenol for pain and Lopressor for high blood pressure. He states he has no allergies.

You remove the soiled bandage to look at the healing incision and note puffiness on the sides of the incision, but no redness or drainage. The skin around the area looks clean and dry. You note that the muscles of the thenar eminence appear atrophied compared to his left hand.

Questions as You Begin

Consider these questions as you begin developing this case:

- How much strength and coordination will Mr. Petrov need in order to continue doing the work on the farm?
- Are there other meaningful roles that he could transition to, letting his son take over more of his physical chores?
- What will happen as they age?
- Should you ask these questions, or is it outside of the scope of your service to him?

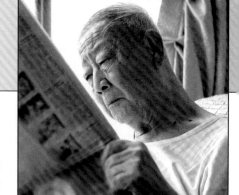

CASE
3.2

CLIENT: John Cho, 74-year-old Asian male

CONDITION: Fractured humerus with ORIF

SETTINGS: Hospital medical/surgical unit; skilled nursing facility

Initial Setting

You have received an occupational therapy referral for John Cho on the medical floor of the hospital where you work. On the referral form you see that he is 74 years old and was admitted to the hospital yesterday with a diagnosis of a fractured right humerus. The referral states "OT for self-care activities and mobilizing unaffected joints of right upper extremity." Before going to the floor to begin his evaluation, you first look for background information in his electronic medical record. On the front sheet it gives Mr. Cho's religion as Buddhist, and lists his race and primary language as Chinese. His health insurance is listed as Medicare and Medicaid. On the admission history and physical report from the admitting physician you see that Mr. Cho was admitted from the emergency department (ED) after his neighbor found him on the floor of his apartment and called the ambulance. From the notes you see that ED staff determined that he had pain in his right arm and hip. He was unable to give much information, but blood work indicated that he had very low blood sugar and was dehydrated. A radiology report taken shortly after he came indicated a displaced fracture of the right humeral head. The report of his right hip did not reveal any fracture. After an initial attempt to realign the fracture through manipulation in the emergency department, it was decided that due to the severity of the displacement, and the patient's inability to follow directions, they would use a surgical procedure with general anesthesia. Mr. Cho was sent to the operating room, where an open reduction with internal fixation (ORIF) was completed successfully, achieving good alignment of the humerus. There was no family with Mr. Cho in the ED, and there was a social work note stating that an attempt was being made to contact the neighbor that called the ambulance to obtain more information. The ED physician recommended admission to the hospital in order to stabilize his blood sugar and monitor the fractured humerus postsurgically, while a discharge plan could be developed. Nursing notes from this morning state that Mr. Cho is trying to communicate with staff, but it is unclear if he is confused or unable to speak much English. He has refused to take several doses of the hydrocodone prescribed for pain, but has allowed nursing staff to give him sliding scale insulin to regulate his blood sugar. He has also had a productive cough since the morning of admission, and the attending physician has ordered a sputum culture. A dietary note indicates Mr. Cho ate very little of his breakfast this morning.

On your way up to the medical floor you notice the social worker, nurse, and dietitian in the staff meeting room discussing this patient, so you join them. The social worker gives an update, telling the care team that he has been in contact with the patient's neighbor, who says Mr. Cho is widowed, has no children and no other family in the area. Mr. Cho speaks fairly good English according to the neighbor, but has been more confused lately. The neighbor knew that Mr. Cho was diabetic, and there were pills in his apartment that he took regularly. The neighbor also shared that it was getting much more difficult for Mr. Cho to take care of his apartment and get groceries. The neighbor wanted to help his friend, but said he was limited in what he could do because he was almost 80 years old himself. The social worker said he had started to explore, with Mr. Cho, the possibilities of discharging him to a skilled nursing facility, but that it would take at least 3 or 4 days to arrange, and that Mr. Cho had become upset during the discussion.

The nurse related that she was able to get a sputum sample from Mr. Cho, and was awaiting the laboratory results. Mr. Cho's blood sugar was still quite unstable on the insulin as ordered, and she was getting in touch with the physician to see if he wanted to make a change in the medication order. The dietitian stated that she was able to communicate with Mr. Cho about his dietary preferences, and was going to adjust his diet in the hope that he would eat more.

When you enter the patient's room, you see that Mr. Cho has a sling supporting his right arm. His right hand appears swollen and black and blue. You can see white gauze covering much of his right upper arm. He is trying to read a newspaper that is lying on his over-bed stand using just his left hand. After you introduce yourself, Mr. Cho answers "hello" appropriately. You ask a few questions and determine that Mr. Cho is oriented to place but not to time. You ask him about some pictures in the newspaper and discover that he enjoys gardening and used to have a dog. Mr. Cho notices the social worker going by the door and points with his left hand, saying, "I don't like him. I will go home."

Questions as You Begin

Consider these questions as you begin developing this case:

- What is Mr. Cho's native language, and would an interpreter be helpful?
- If he is determined to go home, but unable to do some instrumental activities of daily living, would he accept having someone come in to help him?
- Will that be enough for him to be safe?
- What kind of transportation does he use to get groceries, and will he be able to use this to come to outpatient rehabilitation after he is discharged?

Transfer to Skilled Nursing Facility

You receive notice that a new patient, John Cho, has been admitted to the skilled nursing facility where you work, and you schedule him to be seen that afternoon. Before he is brought to the rehabilitation room you review his admission information in the medical chart. The admission coordinator's note indicates that Mr. Cho meets the requirements for skilled care and will be covered for rehabilitation under Medicare Part A for up to 100 days. On the admission and screening information you see that he was admitted to your facility from a hospital, following a fall that resulted in a fractured humerus with ORIF and a bruised hip. While in the hospital for 4 days Mr. Cho was diagnosed with pneumonia, and his blood sugar was unstable. The discharge plan from the hospital indicates that nursing home placement was recommended for further rehabilitation, since he lived alone and was weak and unable to manage his insulin and medications independently. With additional rehabilitation it was thought that he could regain his strength and learn to manage his health and personal care needs in order to return to his apartment in the city, with community services if needed.

The discharge note from the OT in the hospital indicates that Mr. Cho was feeding himself at the time of discharge using his left, nondominant hand with setup and adaptive equipment, and he needed minimal assistance to bathe his upper body. Maximum assistance was needed for lower body bathing, and there was no mention of his level of independence for toileting. The PT discharge note said that he was walking with a quad cane and supervision, and needed cueing for posture and safe transfers. The nursing note mentioned that his blood sugar still needed to be watched carefully and he was discharged to the nursing facility on 5 units of Humalog before meals and 25 units of Lantus before sleep to manage his diabetes, and oral Levaquin for the resolving pneumonia. The nursing discharge note stated that he seemed to understand more English than they had thought at first. At time of discharge he was noted to be oriented to person, place, and time. One of the goals of admitting Mr. Cho to the skilled facility was to see if he could learn to administer his own insulin. The social work note indicated that it had been determined that Mr. Cho spoke Mandarin fluently, and that he had immigrated to the United States in the 1950s as a young man. He had worked as a tailor for a clothing firm in the city for many years. There were no family members listed, but there was a note in the skilled nursing facility's admission records that a friend, Mr. Thompson, had called the facility and said he would like to visit once Mr. Cho was settled.

Mr. Cho was brought to the rehabilitation department in a wheelchair by the activities director. He was wearing a hospital gown and socks. He did not make eye contact at first, and sat quietly in the chair, with a sad expression. His right arm was in a sling, and his right hand had a large area of ecchymosis. The activities director stated that she had learned from Mr. Cho that he enjoyed board games, puzzles, and gardening. After introducing yourself and explaining a little about OT, you ask him why he looks sad. "I don't want to be here," he says, "If I stay too long I will lose my apartment."

Questions as You Begin

Consider these questions as you begin developing this case:

- Why isn't Mr. Cho dressed?
- Is there something that occupational therapy can do to help nursing in training Mr. Cho to manage his diabetes?
- Can the friend, Mr. Thompson, be involved to help Mr. Cho, either psychologically or otherwise?
- How is Mr. Cho's apartment set up? If you know this, how can it help you?

CASE

3.3

CLIENT: Tyler Babcock, 7-year-old African
               American male

CONDITION: Upper extremity amputation

SETTINGS: Hospital inpatient surgical unit;
               outpatient rehabilitation department

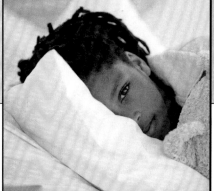

Initial Setting

The O'Donnel Health center is a large medical complex that includes a regional trauma center and a full complement of inpatient services. You work in the Rehabilitation Services Department and are assigned to the orthopedic and surgical floors. Today you have received several new referrals. Most of them are standard joint replacements, but you notice you also have a 7-year-old African American boy named Tyler Babcock who has suffered an upper extremity amputation on your list. You always start your day by gathering information on your new patients, and you log onto your computer to find out about Tyler first.

Tyler was admitted through the emergency department (ED) 3 days ago to Dr. Li Ming's service, a vascular surgeon on staff. From the demographic page you see that Tyler's mother is listed as the custodial parent. Spanish is his primary language, but it was noted that he also speaks English. According to the history and physical in the file, Tyler was healthy and had normal development prior to this incident. On the morning of admission to the hospital, Tyler had gone with some friends and one of his older brothers and was being pulled behind a boat on an inner tube when he was ejected from it along with another child. Although he was wearing a life preserver, he was run over by the boat. His injuries included a partially amputated right arm below the elbow, multiple lacerations, two broken ribs, and a concussion. The people on the boat retrieved both boys from the water, called the coast guard, and tried to provide first aid to Tyler's injuries. He was airlifted from the scene to a trauma center where it was determined that his right arm had suffered so much damage that limb reattachment could not be attempted. Dr. Li Ming performed the surgery to complete the amputation and close the injury. According to the operating room report, the damaged right ulna and radius were shortened leaving approximately 6 in below the elbow, and skin flaps were used to provide a good covering to the remaining forearm.

Tyler has been in the intensive care unit for the past 2 days where he was medically stabilized. You learn that the physician is preparing to move him to the surgical unit in the next 24 hours, and is requesting occupational therapy to begin rehabilitation today. After reviewing the nursing notes you see Tyler has begun talking, and does not appear to have suffered any permanent cognitive deficits from the concussion. According to the initial social work note, Tyler lives with his mother and three older siblings. His mother is Dominican American and speaks Spanish in the home. Tyler is in the first grade. His mother and oldest brother have been staying at the hospital with Tyler, but his mother has been very reluctant to speak with staff. The social worker has been successful in helping her begin the process of enrolling Tyler and his siblings in the federal Children's Health Insurance Program (CHIP).

Later in the morning, you go to the intensive care unit and discover that Tyler was moved a half hour ago to an inpatient surgical unit. You find him in a private room with his mother and brother. He is sitting up in bed with his right upper extremity supported on pillows. You notice that the injured residual limb is wrapped in an elastic compression dressing. Tyler's family members are speaking quietly in Spanish when you enter, but stop speaking when they see you. You introduce yourself and explain what occupational therapy is. Then you tell Tyler that you will be helping him with using his left arm for things like dressing and eating. His older brother speaks up: "I thought they said he'd be getting an artificial arm." You explain that it takes a while for that, and meanwhile it is best if Tyler becomes as independent as possible.

Questions as You Begin

Consider these questions as you begin developing this case:

- How has the psychological trauma of this amputation affected Tyler and his family?
- How can you relate to a 7-year-old in this kind of situation?
- His family seems very close and somewhat protective. How should you deal with this when it comes to Tyler's therapy?
- You know some Spanish. Would it be helpful to use it to establish a relationship with Tyler and his family?
- Or would that be considered rude to use a little Spanish if you don't speak it fluently?

Transfer to Outpatient Rehabilitation

You work in a busy outpatient clinic that is part of a large medical complex along with many doctors' offices, a phlebotomy station, radiology service, and an oncology treatment center as well as a small, day-surgery center. Many of the specialists in the center have privileges at area hospitals and specialty medical centers. You have received a referral from Dr. Li Ming, a vascular surgeon who has offices in the complex. He has requested occupational therapy for a young patient of his who suffered a traumatic amputation as a result of a boating accident. A lot of information was faxed over to your office about this young patient's history, course of recovery, and early assessments and treatment. You sit down to review the information and find out about Tyler Babcock.

Tyler is a 7-year-old African American male. He suffered a partial below-elbow amputation of his right upper extremity in a boating accident. The amputation was completed surgically when the limb could not be saved. Nursing and physician notes indicate that Tyler recovered well following the surgery, with stable vital signs, no residual cognitive deficits, and good healing of his many lacerations. You learn that he stayed in the intensive care unit for 2 days before being moved out onto the surgical floors. He began showing some signs of infection at the surgical site on day 5 of his admission, and was started on an antibiotic. Edema in his residual limb was measurably decreased 2 days later when he was discharged, with the skin assessment noting an improvement in the skin integrity over the surgical area. Tyler was doing fairly well with keeping his right upper extremity elevated and doing active range of motion of the elbow with prompting.

The hospital social work note added context about Tyler's support system and home environment. He is in the first grade at a local public school, and receives average grades. Tyler lives with his mother and three older brothers in an older residential area outside this mid-sized city. His father has had no contact with the family over the past 5 years. Tyler's mother works as a clerk at a local department store, and she is very active in the Catholic Church in her community, taking the children regularly. She emigrated as a young adult from the Dominican Republic and speaks Spanish as her primary language. She gained US citizenship after marrying an American, also of Dominican descent. All of her children were born in the United States, and the children are fluent in both Spanish and English. Tyler has just been approved for health insurance through CHIP for low-income families. Social work notes indicate that his mother and older brother visited Tyler frequently in the hospital, but were reluctant to speak with staff.

Tyler and his mother were shown how to massage his residual limb in the hospital and apply wraps to form the "cone" shaped stump in preparation for a prosthesis. Tyler was in the hospital for a total of 7 days before being discharged home to his family. Nursing notes show that he was fitted with a shrinker sock on the day before discharge to decrease postoperative edema and continue forming the stump. A prosthetist also made a preliminary visit to begin the measuring process, but would not be able to fabricate an initial prosthesis until the healing had progressed further and more shrinkage had occurred. The occupational therapist note stated she worked with Tyler in the hospital on transferring hand dominance and performing basic ADLs one-handed; however, she had a difficult time getting him to engage. At discharge he still needed a great deal of encouragement with toileting and dressing tasks using his left hand. He was independent in feeding except for cutting his food. Grip and pinch strength in his left, nondominant hand was listed in the OT discharge summary as within normal limits. His interests were listed as playing board games, and at home he also liked riding his bike and playing with the family pets. Upon discharge he was receiving Tylenol with codeine to control pain, as well as Keflex to address his infection.

The social work discharge note mentions that there had been no visitors other than his mother and brothers, and Tyler's mother seemed to be overwhelmed at the prospect of taking him home. Referrals were made for outpatient therapy to continue after discharge, both preprosthetic and postprosthetic. Today's initial outpatient visit was 3 days after his discharge from the hospital.

Tyler and his mother arrive promptly for his appointment to therapy. She completes the required paperwork without asking any questions. When you introduce yourself, Tyler does not make eye contact, but his mother responds to your greeting and encourages her son to do the same. You invite both of them to accompany you back to the treatment area. Tyler has a long-sleeved shirt on, with the right cuff tucked into his jeans pocket. You notice that he keeps the elbow of the residual right limb flexed at about 45 degrees. You begin by asking both of them how things have been going since Tyler returned home a few days ago. His mother states she is worried whether his arm is healing properly and that she does not want the doctor to be upset with her when he has a follow-up visit in a few days. She also tells you that Tyler has been having some problems with urinary incontinence since returning home.

When you ask Tyler simple questions, he either shrugs or answers with one word. You give him a marker and a puzzle page and encourage him to try it, and he picks the marker up with his left hand. When you ask what he likes to play at home, he answers, "Xbox!" His mother adds that he also likes to play with their two dogs and ride his bike. When you ask him to remove his shrinker sock and bandages he turns to his mother and holds out his injured right upper extremity for her assistance. His mother explains that Tyler has been very dependent on his family to help him, and he is left alone with his brothers when she works in the evening. She doesn't know what she will do for childcare when his siblings are at school and she works. You ask about Tyler returning to school, but she simply says, "He can't! He's not ready! He needs help toileting and eating. He can't do anything for himself yet."

Questions as You Begin

Consider these questions as you begin developing this case:

- Can school, or his school friends be instrumental in helping motivate Tyler to get involved with normal activities again?
- What could be causing the urinary incontinence?
- Are his older siblings and mother doing too much for him, interfering with his independence?
- How can you help the family reestablish a healthy routine for Tyler until he returns to school?
- You have little to no experience working with someone with an upper extremity amputation. Should you hand this case off to a more experienced therapist?

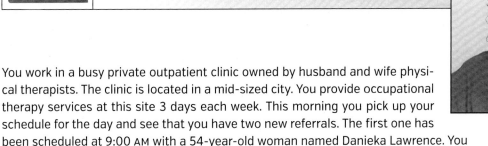

CASE

3.4

CLIENT: Danieka Lawrence, 54-year-old African American female

CONDITION: Lateral epicondylitis

SETTING: Private outpatient rehabilitation clinic

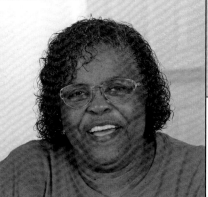

You work in a busy private outpatient clinic owned by husband and wife physical therapists. The clinic is located in a mid-sized city. You provide occupational therapy services at this site 3 days each week. This morning you pick up your schedule for the day and see that you have two new referrals. The first one has been scheduled at 9:00 AM with a 54-year-old woman named Danieka Lawrence. You retrieve the file that has been started for the client to see what information you can learn prior to her arrival. A local orthopedist, Dr. Daniel Watson has referred this client and provided both a script and a brief history. In addition, the secretary for your clinic made notes on the intake form from her conversation with the client when she set up the appointment.

From these sources you glean the following information: Danieka Lawrence is a 54-year-old Jamaican immigrant, living in an apartment complex in the city. She makes a living by running a childcare service out of her apartment. She lives with her husband and one teen-aged daughter, and has two older children still in Jamaica. Her husband works as a mechanic. Danieka has Blue Cross–Blue Shield insurance through her husband's employer. The client went to the physician complaining of right elbow pain 4 weeks ago. The client's medical history and physical revealed that she has an irregular heart rate treated with Cardizem and Coumadin. Dr. Watson diagnosed the elbow pain as lateral epicondylitis and prescribed nonsteroidal anti-inflammatory drugs (NSAIDs) and a counterforce brace. One week ago the client made a follow-up visit to the doctor and complained that the pain had not improved. Dr. Watson administered a Cortisone shot to the right elbow joint and recommended therapy.

Danieka Lawrence arrives several minutes late to the clinic for her appointment with you. She is a heavy woman, very friendly and outgoing, and speaks English with a strong accent. She tells you that she had a difficult time getting someone to cover her at home to watch the children, so she is concerned about how she is going to be able to come regularly for therapy. She tells you to call her "Dani." Once you take seats in the exam room of the clinic, you ask her to tell you about the elbow pain. She rates her elbow pain as a 5 out of 10 most of the time, but 8 or 9 out of 10 when she uses her right arm. She also says the Cortisone shot does not seem to have helped. When you inquire about the circumstances that seem to make the pain worse, she describes lifting the children, pulling the trash bag out of the can, and carrying groceries. When asked about anything that has helped reduce the pain, she says not using it and ice. She expresses concern that she has to use her arms regularly for lifting, so she is not sure how she is going to recover. She also adds confidentially that she is worried about being reported because her business is all "under the table." While talking about activities, you ask her what she does to relax. With a smile she says, "Baking and sewing!"

Questions as You Begin

Consider these questions as you begin developing this case:

- How can Mrs. Lawrence reduce her repetitive stress activities and still engage in important activities?
- Can the husband and daughter help in some way?
- If the counterforce brace and Cortisone shot did not help, what clues does that give you?
- Should you be concerned that this client is running a childcare program without a license?
- What is your responsibility, now that she has told you this?

CASE

3.5

CLIENT: Yelina Lopez Moreno, 36-year-old Hispanic female

CONDITION: Colles fracture with ORIF

SETTING: Hospital outpatient rehabilitation clinic

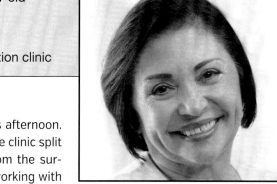

Yelina Lopez Moreno is scheduled to see you for an evaluation this afternoon. Your outpatient clinic is part of a nonprofit hospital. Therapists in the clinic split their time between seeing hospital inpatients and outpatients from the surrounding rural community. Today you were very busy all morning working with inpatients and finally sit down to do some paperwork and have a bite to eat before the outpatients start arriving. You see that you are scheduled for mostly revisits with one new evaluation as your first appointment this afternoon. Yelina Lopez Mareno was referred for Occupational Therapy by an orthopedic surgeon that works for the hospital, whom you know quite well. The referral form, however, gives you very little information. Other than the client's name you see that your new client is a 36-year-old female. The diagnosis is listed as a right Colles fracture status post open reduction and internal fixation (ORIF). Although her private insurance is listed, you note that treatment will be covered by Worker's Compensation through her employer.

You know that you can get more information through the electronic medical record system that is linked to the physician offices, so you log onto your computer to do a search. A review of the demographic records in the electronic record system reveals that the client is listed as Hispanic, and Spanish is her primary language. Her occupation is listed as nurse's aide. Her next of kin is listed as her sister, and you note that she lives on a rural route outside of town. Her marital status is divorced, and her religious affiliation is Catholic. Next you review the most recent history and physical on your client. Her history is unremarkable with no chronic disorders other than gastroesophageal reflux disease (GERD) for which she takes Prilosec. She has had three natural pregnancies without complications. She has had no previous surgeries, fractures, or musculoskeletal conditions prior to her current diagnosis. The history states that the fracture of her right distal radius and ulna occurred in the nursing home where she works. She told the physician that she put her hand out to stop a door from slamming on a resident. Not only did the door slam into her outstretched hand, but her hand was then trapped in the door as it closed. She was brought to the emergency room for an x-ray, which revealed compound fractures of both long bones of her forearm. The orthopedist on call decided that surgery would be needed to achieve good alignment of the bone fragments and to repair the soft-tissue damage.

The operating room report shows that an open reduction was performed the day after the injury and a plate and screws were used to fix the bones with good results. A cast was applied following surgery and she was prescribed Vicodin for pain. The physician's office note states that satisfactory healing was noted at 4 weeks and 6 weeks postsurgery. The cast was removed at 6 weeks and the client was referred for therapy. You note from the date of injury that your client is now almost 7 weeks postsurgery.

Mrs. Martinez arrives a few minutes early for her appointment and completes the paperwork as requested. You observe that she is dressed in jeans and a sweater, and is accompanied by a Hispanic woman of about the same age. You introduce yourself, and Mrs. Martinez smiles and turns to the woman sitting next to her. The woman introduces herself as Mrs. Martinez's sister, Maria. She tells you that she has driven the client to therapy today, and that she will be happy to translate, as Yelina understands English fairly well but needs some assistance at times with communicating, especially if she is nervous. You know the hospital's policy is to use certified translators when necessary, so you are not sure what to do. You offer to arrange for a translator but both Yelina and her sister shake their heads "no," insisting they don't need one. Maria explains that her English is very good, and Yelina would not be comfortable with someone else. Yelina says, "Yes, please." Maria invites you to call them both by their first names.

You welcome them to the clinic and ask them to come back to the treatment area. You begin the assessment by asking to see Yelina's injured arm and you ask your client how she has been feeling since the cast was removed. Yelina indicates she understands by pulling up the arm of her sweater and holding her right arm out and saying, "hurts very much." You notice that her forearm and hand appear quite swollen. The incisions are dry and edges are well approximated. There is some dried blood and eschar noted, but no evidence of infection. When you ask if the Vicodin helps reduce the pain, she says, "So-so." You ask her about rest and sleep and she tells you through Maria that she sleeps poorly, most times just staying on the couch for the night. You ask her to show you if she can move her fingers on her right hand, and she moves all of her digits a few degrees, and grimaces. Maria confirms that Yelina is right-hand dominant.

Next, you ask Yelina how she uses her hands at work and at home. With the help of her sister you learn that Yelina works full time as a nurse's aide at a skilled nursing facility. She does a lot of heavy lifting throughout the course of her shift. At home she has three children to care for, aged 8, 14, and 17. Her time is filled with cooking, cleaning, and laundry. She usually drives herself, but hasn't been able to since her accident. Maria looks fondly at her sister and tells you, "It has been hard on my sister. I'm worried that she is getting depressed. She has had some problems with depression before, but she isn't taking any medicine for it now." Maria suggests that the best thing for Yelena will be if she can return to work as soon as it is safe to do so. Yelina does not look happy about this suggestion. You wonder whether Yelina wants to return to her job, and you ask her directly. She answers in Spanish and her sister translates reluctantly. "She says she has to keep this job so she and her children will have health insurance. She hopes she can continue to be off work as long as possible with this injury." When you ask what she enjoys doing when she has some time to herself, she says cooking and watching television, especially soap operas on Spanish television.

Questions as You Begin

Consider these questions as you begin developing this case:

- You wonder if depression is affecting Yelina's desire to reengage in activities again. Or does she just not like her job very much?
- Should you suggest that she talk to her primary care physician or mental health counselor about her depression in light of this injury?
- Her sister seems very close to Yelina. Is there some way that she can be involved in therapy? Or would that make Yelina more dependent?

CASE
3.6

CLIENT:	Glen Hobart, 56-year-old Caucasian male
CONDITION:	Flexor tendon repair
SETTINGS:	Hospital inpatient surgical unit; outpatient rehabilitation clinic

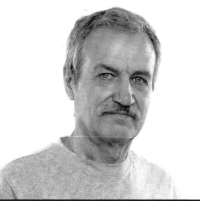

Initial Setting

Mercy General Hospital is located in the middle of a densely populated urban area. You work in the rehabilitation department and share your time between seeing patients in the hospital and working with the transitional care unit that is part of the facility. Yesterday afternoon at the daily team meeting on the medical/surgical unit of the hospital, you were told that there was a new man admitted who had suffered a serious tendon laceration. You were not surprised to see the referral for the new patient with the tendon repair on your desk when you came in this morning. After completing morning treatments with your patients on the transitional care unit, you sit down to learn as much as you can about the new referral.

The referral form gives the patient's name as Glen Hobart, a 56-year-old Caucasian male. His diagnosis is listed as laceration of the right flexor tendon in zone III, status post repair of flexor digitorum superficialis. There was also a note in the comment section of the referral form that the client was hearing-impaired, but reads lips well, and can make himself understood fairly easily. You decide to go up on the floor to access the medical chart in order to gather more information prior to seeing the patient. At the nurses' station, you locate Mr. Hobart's chart and turn first to the face sheet for more demographic information. Mr. Hobart's wife is listed as the next of kin, and he has private insurance through his job at a local bank. Next, you turn to the admission section of the chart. You see that he was admitted through the emergency department (ED) where he was taken after an incident that occurred at home while he was doing some carpentry work. The patient was reported to have suffered a deep cut to the palm of his dominant right hand while working with a table saw. In the ED, he was given a tetanus shot and X-ray images were taken of his injured hand. Although the report came back with no fractured bones in his hand, it was determined that the deep laceration would likely need surgical repair of the underlying soft-tissue damage. An orthopedic surgeon with a hand specialty was called in and further assessment of the injury was conducted. Assessment of active flexion for each digit indicated a need to repair flexor digitorum superficialis but not flexor digitorum profundus for at least two digits on the patient's right hand. After testing with 2-point discrimination, it was determined that there was no concurrent nerve damage. A nursing note indicates that Mr. Hobart was assisted with communication in the ED by his wife and teenaged daughter, but that he was able to participate through lip reading and some speech.

The operating room report shows that Mr. Hobart underwent primary surgical repair of the flexor digitorum superficialis tendons for digits 2, 3, and 4 early the next morning. Each of these three tendons was noted during the operation to be completely severed, but viable for direct tendon repair. The tendon to digit 5 was less than 25% severed, and it was decided not to repair this tendon in order to minimize the potential for complications from the repair itself. The flexor digitorum profundus as it crosses through the same area was visualized during the operation and determined to be spared from injury. There were no significant neurovascular injuries noted during the repair. The postoperative note documented good postsurgical recovery of blood flow to all digits with good approximation of the edges of the laceration. A bulky dressing was applied to position the right wrist and metacarpophalangeal joints in flexion, and interphalangeal joints in extension. Postoperatively, the surgeon recommended the Kleinert treatment protocol with early mobility and a dorsal blocking splint.

In the medical history and physical section of the medical record, you note that the client has a history of back pain treated with Percocet, and a history of gout managed with Colchicine. Mr. Hobart had no other medical or surgical issues noted, and no allergies. The physician's progress note anticipated a 1- to 2-day hospital stay followed by outpatient therapy following the Kleinert protocol to regain the use of his hand. In the social work note on admission, you find some additional information related to the client's personal context. Mr. Hobart has a Master's degree in Business Administration from a large university. He has three teenaged children who live at home with him and his wife. None of the other members of his family are hearing-impaired, but all can sign. Their home is in one of the newer suburbs. His wife works in the same bank that he does, and the social worker notes that Mr. Hobart is very anxious to minimize his time away from work. His leisure interests are carpentry and lawn care.

After your chart review, you go back to the rehabilitation clinic to get some information on the Kleinert protocol. You notice that there is a Duran protocol and a modified Duran protocol in the same file. After returning to the floor, you proceed to Mr. Hobart's room. You knock on his closed door but don't hear any response. You open his door and announce who you are, proceeding into the lit room. Once inside, you see Mr. Hobart sitting in the bedside chair and looking at a laptop on the over-bed stand. He glances up noticing you and smiles, beckoning you to enter with his unbandaged hand and then closes his computer. You introduce yourself, making a conscious effort to enunciate. He extends his left hand to shake awkwardly, pointing to the bandage on his right hand and shaking his head. He attempts to make some signs with his left hand, but you tell him apologetically that you don't understand sign language. He begins to speak slowly. "Hi, I'm Glen and I'm glad you are going to help me. What do you want me to do?" You tell him you would like to have a sign language interpreter join you for the initial evaluation. He shrugs and says "Okay." After telling him that you will be back shortly, you go to the nursing station and ask for the contact information for the on-call interpreter. Fortunately, he was available and had already met Mr. Hobart, so he was able to join you for the evaluation. You begin by asking Mr. Hobart how he used his hands at work. Mostly typing or writing? "Mostly signing!" he laughs, "my wife is my boss and we talk a lot."

Questions as You Begin

Consider these questions as you begin developing this case:

- Since the surgeon has specified the Kleinert protocol, should you discuss alternatives such as Duran or Modified Duran with him because they are newer?
- You are concerned about creating a splint for him so soon after the injury. How can you fabricate this as efficiently and with as little stress to his injured hand as possible?
- You have never worked with someone that is deaf before, and the interpreter is very busy. Should you try the next session without the interpreter?
- How is the loss of the use of his right hand going to affect his ability to communicate with friends and family?

Transfer to Outpatient Rehabilitation

At the end of a busy day, you sit down at your desk to look at tomorrow's schedule. You are assigned to the outpatient services of the rehabilitation department at Mercy General Hospital. You see that you have a new referral for a patient that was just discharged from the inpatient unit after undergoing a flexor tendon repair to his right hand. You are sure he must have received occupational therapy services before he left the hospital, so you log onto the computer to find background information on this referral.

After reading the medical history and physical and the operating room report, you turn to the therapy notes. You see that your colleague Jody provided treatment for Mr. Hobart for his brief 2-day inpatient stay. Her treatment included fabrication of a Kleinert splint with dynamic digit flexion. She had instructed the patient in active extension exercises with the splint in place to prevent full extension at the metacarpophalangeal (mcp) joints of the involved fingers. She had also recommended several pieces of adaptive equipment to help him with one-handed ADLs during his recovery.

You notice that Jody is at her desk on the other side of the clinic and decide to get some additional information about Mr. Hobart. You are surprised to learn that Mr. Hobart is hearing-impaired, because you had not noticed this in his chart. You are concerned about being able to communicate adequately with your new client and ask if you should arrange for an interpreter, but Jody assures you that she found she really hadn't needed the interpreter during her evaluation. She also tells you that Mrs. Hobart is herself a trained interpreter, and will accompany him to therapy on the first day. You also learn that Mr. Hobart is very anxious to return to his job, and is diligent in following all recommendations. "In fact," she tells you, "you have to watch him carefully because he has a tendency to overdo."

The next day, Glen Hobart is your first patient. He arrives early with his wife and completes the forms with no difficulty. The reception staff escorts them to the treatment area where you meet him for the initial evaluation. With the help of his wife, Mr. Hobart tells you that he has been careful not to bump his hand or get the dressing wet, and he has been doing his exercises regularly. You discover that if you listen carefully, you are able to understand most of what he says, although you are glad that his wife is there to translate at least during the initial evaluation. You look at his hand and note that it seems to be healing well, with no signs of infection and only a small amount of swelling in the back of the hand and digits. You review his home program with him, and his wife tells you, "Yesterday he did too much and then his hand was incredibly swollen for the rest of the day." "You have to understand," Mr. Hobart jokes, "I'm home with three teenagers and I am going crazy. I have to get back to work."

Questions as You Begin

Consider these questions as you begin developing this case:

- You notice from reading through the protocol that full recovery will take quite a while, and Mr. Hobart is really anxious to get back to work. What can you do to keep his motivation for work from interfering with his recovery?
- Is there a way to reestablish his normal routines and patterns, even if he cannot return to his job yet?
- Does having his wife as his supervisor at work complicate things?
- If so, what can you do about it?

CLIENT: Thomas Carducci, 58-year-old
                 Caucasian male

CONDITION: Total hip replacement

SETTING: Hospital inpatient orthopedic unit

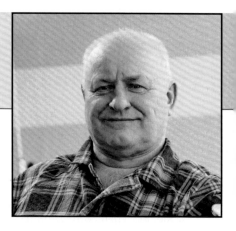

St. Mark's hospital is a large for-profit healthcare provider. You work in the inpatient rehabilitation department of the acute care center, and are adjacent to the surgical floor. Today, you will be seeing clients with a variety of orthopedic conditions. Typically, you will work with them in their hospital rooms for the first day or two, and if they are in the hospital longer than that, you will bring them down to the rehabilitation clinic for additional treatment. You see that you have a new evaluation for a patient named Thomas Carducci, a 58-year-old male with a diagnosis of osteoarthritis, status post total hip replacement. You note from the patient's information on the referral note that he is 5 feet 10 inches tall and 368 pounds.

The electronic medical record allows you to find additional information on your patients, and you open the record to learn more about Mr. Carducci. In the demographic data, you discover that he is married and lists his wife as next of kin, and lists Catholic as his religion. He works for a gas company and has private insurance through his company. The history and physical section indicates that Mr. Carducci has type 2 diabetes controlled with Metformin. He has a long history of joint pain in his knees and hips, and takes Naproxen Sodium routinely to manage this pain. He has had a Cortisone shot in his right hip previously, which helped for about 3 months. The physician notes that previous attempts by the patient to lose weight have been unsuccessful. You note in the operating room report that Mr. Carducci underwent a metal on metal implant to replace his right femoral head and acetabulum. He was reported to have good alignment achieved with the prosthesis and his recovery after surgery was unremarkable. He was started on Vicodin for pain after surgery and was given an ice-water pad to manage the edema around his right hip. In the discharge planning section, it is anticipated that Mr. Carducci will be in the hospital for 3 days following surgery, and will return home with his wife and a referral for homecare services.

There is a social work note on the chart as well as a completed physical therapy note from earlier today. In the social work intake note, the patient's home is described as a ranch, with three steps to enter. The husband's wife is a school teacher who plans to take a week off from work when her husband returns home. The couple has five children and a large extended family in the area. There is one son still living at home and going to a local college. Mr. Carducci is off of work temporarily and plans to return to work once his physician states that he is fully recovered for his job as a supervisor for gas line installation. The note also indicates that Mr. Carducci's wife is a small woman and has expressed concern about her ability to assist her husband if he is not able to get around on his own when he is discharged. The physical therapy assessment notes that following surgery the patient was cooperative with ankle pumps and heel slides while supine, but refused to attempt standing or moving to the bedside chair due to pain. Transfer recommendations at this time were listed as use of stand assist device and two-person assist due to Mr. Carducci's size to avoid injury to the patient or staff until physical therapy can work with him again this afternoon and further evaluate his status.

Before closing the record and going up to see the patient, you notice that a note has been entered by the dietitian. You read through it and notice she has said that Mr. Carducci is uncooperative and refusing the recommended diabetic diet. The dietitian has a plan to offer nutrition and diabetic counseling for the patient and his wife while in the hospital.

Nursing notes reflect relatively stable vital signs, frequent requests for additional pain medication, and food requests. The skin assessments note that the incision is showing no signs of infection, edges are well approximated, and standard hip precautions have been reviewed with the patient. His blood sugar levels have been variable, and nursing notes that they plan to speak with the patient's primary physician and the surgeon about recommendations to bring his blood sugar levels under better control.

After gathering some basic assessment materials you find the client's room and knock on the door. You hear a brusk "come in!" and enter. In the private room, you find the client reclined in bed with the television on and a roomful of people, including two young children. After introducing yourself, you discover that the visitors include the patient's wife, three of his children with their spouses, and two grandchildren. You notice several containers of food on the over-bed stand and on the window sill that appear to have been brought in by the family. You explain to Mr. Carducci that you need to complete an initial assessment with him. All of the visitors except his wife decide it is time to leave. Mr. Carducci does not appear pleased by this development and tries to change their minds, saying "This will only take a couple of minutes 'cause I can't really do anything yet." After they leave you start by asking Mr. Carducci to tell you about his work and leisure activities so that you understand his occupational performance goals. He quickly explains that his job is very physical, so when he gets home he is too tired to do much more than watch television or read before dinner. When asked to share some more about his job, he relates that he is an inspector for the gas company, so he drives to multiple sites every day to check on jobs. You comment on how good his room smells and his wife smiles shyly. "I know I probably shouldn't," she says, "but if I didn't bring Tommy his favorite Italian food, he would think I didn't love him!" "Yeah," Tommy says, "can you tell we're just a little Italian? You have to try some of these stuffed shells!"

Questions as You Begin

Consider these questions as you begin developing this case:

- You find yourself feeling angry about Mr. Carducci's lack of compliance with diet and therapy. You are concerned that your feelings may interfere with therapy, and decide you had better get a grip on them so that you will be able to develop a therapeutic relationship with him. As you think about what the cause of these feelings might be, you wonder, are you biased against people who are obese?
- He has undoubtedly been warned by his doctor before about the consequences of his lifestyle on his health, so hearing it from you probably won't change anything. What is he motivated by?
- What role does his cultural background play in his health management?
- How can you deal with any personal biases you may have?

Chronic Musculoskeletal Conditions

Treatment of chronic musculoskeletal conditions is provided across all levels of care. Given its chronic nature, most (but not all) clients with these conditions will be middle-aged to elderly in years. Although two of the four cases presented are limited in the scope of the condition (trigger finger and Dupuytren's contracture) arthritis, both osteo- and rheumatoid type, can impact multiple aspects of a person's performance. Consider the older woman who is living alone, and suffers from years of chronic rheumatoid arthritis. It probably disrupts her ability to sleep comfortably, dress and bathe easily, prepare meals, and drive. You may be able to improve her quality of life for a long time by helping her find methods of pain management and educating her about joint protection and compensatory techniques that will allow her to remain independent. When a client like this comes into the hospital for an acute condition such as a cardiopulmonary incident, trying to help her participate in a rehabilitation program will be complicated by the comorbidity of rheumatoid arthritis. At the other end of the continuum of care, staff at the residential skilled nursing facility will certainly need to address the impact of chronic musculoskeletal conditions on function to help their clients maintain their performance at whatever level is possible.

As therapists, clients with severe chronic musculoskeletal conditions can be complex if there are multiple joints involved, especially if disease management involves making significant lifestyle changes. Since many of these clients are older, they are more likely to have such complicating factors as diabetes, impaired eyesight and sensory conditions, or impaired memory. However, clients we treat with such chronic conditions can also be some of the most satisfying clients to work with, because of the satisfaction that comes from having such a significant impact on someone's life, with conditions that they may have struggled with for years.

CASE 3.8	CLIENT:	Sylvia Carter, 78-year-old Caucasian female
	CONDITION:	Rheumatoid arthritis
	SETTINGS:	Private outpatient rehabilitation clinic, homecare agency

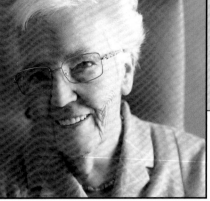

Initial Setting

You have a light schedule today and are in the rehabilitation office at Quality One Rehabilitation Clinic catching up on paperwork. The department's secretary, Linda, approaches you with a concerned look on her face. "Can you possibly see a new evaluation?" she asks. You are surprised when she hesitantly adds, "Now?" When you ask her to explain, she tells you that Miss Carter was confused about the schedule and came on the wrong day. This client had a difficult time making transportation arrangements, Linda explains, and was really hoping to be seen today as long as she was already here. "She said she would be happy to wait if she needs to." You sigh and agree to see her. You know that the other staff would have helped if they were the one with room on their schedule. After asking Linda to tell the new client that it would be a few minutes, you begin looking for information in the electronic medical record system to prepare for the evaluation.

You work in a privately owned rehabilitation clinic in a mid-sized city. Most days you have a full schedule, seeing new revisits every half hour. Evaluations are usually scheduled for 45 minutes, and you typically try to complete the paperwork directly into the computerized system as you go. You pull up the background information on your new client.

Sylvia Carter is a 78-year-old Caucasian female with a long history of rheumatoid arthritis. She is listed as single and gives a nephew's name as a contact person. Her insurance is listed as Medicare Part A and B. Her religious affiliation is Methodist. The referral is from Dr. Patel, her primary physician, who notes that she has multiple joint deformities. A note attached by Dr. Patel states that Miss Carter is a retired librarian. She has no cognitive impairment and lives alone, but is having difficulty caring for herself. Lately she has been having episodes of anxiety, and her relatives and physician are questioning whether she is able to safely remain at home independently. Dr. Patel asks you to explore "remediation and/or adaptive equipment to enhance independence."

The history and physical are unremarkable other than the rheumatoid arthritis. You notice that she is on Toradol and Prednisone for the arthritis, and a few vitamins but no other medication. She had her tonsils out as a child, and a hysterectomy when she was in her fifties. She has no allergies. Miss Carter lives alone in a large old Victorian house in an older neighborhood near the center of town.

You use the intercom to reach Linda and ask her to bring Miss Carter back to meet you in the first evaluation room. You watch the client as she walks slowly using a quad cane in her left hand. She has a pocketbook over her right arm. She is a small, neatly dressed woman with stooped shoulders. When Linda introduces you, Miss Carter clasps your hand in both of hers. She thanks you for fitting her into your schedule. Once seated, you explain what the referral was for, and ask her about her ability to use her hands. She shakes her head and holds out both hands to show you the deformed joints. You note multiple swan neck deformities in both hands as well as "Z" thumb deformities. When you ask about her pain, she says she has gotten used to all her joints aching, but her biggest concern is the loss of strength in her hands. "It's gotten so it takes me an hour just to get dressed – and that's with elastic waistbands, too!" Then she bends closer and lowers her voice. "If I can't take care of myself, I think they'll send me to a home!" You smile at her continuing to hold her fragile hands. "Let's see what we can do if we work together," you reply. As you work through the initial evaluation, you find out that Sylvia Carter has never married, is a retired school librarian, and has helped as a literacy volunteer through the public library after she retired, until she could no longer drive a year ago. At home, she continues to enjoy looking things up on the computer. Miss Carter answers all of your questions quietly, and is very willing to participate in the assessment.

Questions as You Begin

Consider these questions as you begin developing this case:

- You realize that you will need to understand her daily routines and habits, and how her home is set up before you can begin making recommendations. What is the best way to do this without making a home visit?
- Miss Carter seems very frail and tires easily during the evaluation. She wants to get her strength back, but you are afraid to give her exercises because that may leave her with less energy to do her other important activities. When you inquire about getting someone to come to the house to help her, Miss Carter becomes very anxious. "I am a very private person. I've never lived with anyone and I don't want a stranger coming in to mess things up in my house!" You are concerned that you have made a mistake. Was it too soon to ask this question?
- How can you restore trust with this client?

Transfer to Homecare

You have just received a referral from a Dr. Patel to provide occupational therapy through the homecare agency you work for to Sylvia Carter, a 78-year-old woman with rheumatoid arthritis resulting in multiple joint deformities in both hands. You see that the physician has attached a discharge summary from a local rehabilitation clinic that has been working with Miss Carter. The summary states that Miss Carter has improved in self-care skills with improved joint mobility, pain management, and use of adaptive equipment. From the occupational therapy discharge summary you can see that the therapist suggested the referral to homecare for a home evaluation and recommendations to further enhance independence in the home. You call the number on the referral and reach Miss Carter right away. An appointment is arranged at her home on the following afternoon.

When you arrive you are surprised at how large the stately old home is. Six steps lead onto a large front porch with a beautiful wooden door. After ringing the bell, you wait a long time for Miss Carter to reach the door. She calls to you through the door and asks you to open it and come in. Once inside she apologizes, and explains that she can no longer work this door handle. You understand once she holds out her hands and you see the multiple severe joint deformities. Miss Carter invites you to come back to the kitchen where she sits on a stool, explaining that it's easier for her to get up from this seat. She asks you if you would like to join her for a cup of tea and you accept, observing how she goes about the task. You note that she is careful to only fill the kettle part way, uses both hands for lifting, and uses plastic insulated mugs with large handles. After she sits again she says, "I hope you can help me as much as that nice young man at the clinic. I want to do everything I can to stay in my home, and I don't want an aide!"

You notice a jigsaw puzzle on a side table in the kitchen and ask Miss Carter about her leisure interests. Miss Carter tells you she used to sew and knit in addition to reading, but now the only thing she can do easily is the jigsaw puzzles and working on the computer, which she describes as her "window on the world." You ask if she is up to showing you around the rooms that she uses, and she replies, "It won't take long–I only use three rooms." As she walks slowly toward the back of the house where her bedroom is you ask her about her sleep routine. She notes that this is a significant problem for her. She finds it hard to undress when she is tired, and the struggle leaves her frustrated, which makes it that much harder to fall asleep. She mentions that the adaptive equipment she worked on in therapy has helped this to some extent.

Questions as You Begin

Consider these questions as you begin developing this case:

- Miss Carter is very sweet, and you are determined to help her, but her house is huge and makes everything harder for her to do. Should you broach the subject of moving to her?
- Several suggestions you make would require moving pieces of furniture or where things are stored. She listens at first, but then dismisses your ideas and insists you just need to help her get stronger. You see she is quickly becoming very anxious. You are not sure how things went so wrong. How can you get the session back on track?

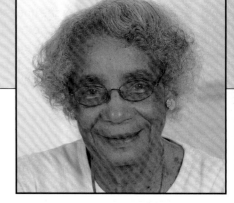

CASE 3.9

CLIENT:	Geraldine Johnson, 65-year-old African American female
CONDITION:	Trigger finger release
SETTING:	Outpatient rehabilitation clinic

The Freeport Health Center is a large orthopedic medical center with a variety of specialties, outpatient surgery center, and various support services. You work in the rehabilitation clinic that provides service to clients of the Health Center. In your clinic you have physical and occupational therapists, some like you who are generalists, and others who have gone on for additional certifications. Your caseload includes a lot of common orthopedic conditions such as carpal tunnel, radial fractures, and epicondylitis. Today, you have a new evaluation with a client diagnosed with trigger finger. You see that this is a postsurgical case, and you look in the medical information system to get some background on this client prior to her initial visit.

The referral is from Dr. Azhir, one of the hand surgeons at the orthopedic center. In the demographic information, you see that the patient is a 65-year-old African American woman named Geraldine Johnson. An admission note from a previous office visit states that she lives with and cares for her ailing mother, and sometimes needs to bring her mother with her when she comes in. She is divorced and has two grown children. Her religious affiliation is Baptist and she is covered by Medicare Part A and B for outpatient services. Under employment status you see that it says "secretary."

The most recent medical history and physical show that Mrs. Johnson has high cholesterol for which she takes Lipitor. Her medical record states that she is "mildly obese" and has difficulty following a healthy diet. She has some osteoarthritis in her left hip and knee and takes over-the-counter anti-inflammatory medication to manage the pain. She has no allergies.

The diagnosis for this referral is listed as right third finger tenosynovitis, status post release. A copy of the recent medical history and physical notes that pain and "triggering" in this finger has been bothering Mrs. Johnson for approximately 1 year. She received a steroid injection several months earlier in the base of her right third finger with no relief. After getting significantly worse recently, Mrs. Johnson spoke with her primary physician and was referred to Dr. Azhir for consideration of a surgical release. In the preoperative report, the physician noted that Mrs. Johnson was a secretary through a temporary service, and was unable to work because of the trigger finger.

Dr. Azhir performed an open release on the client's right third digit, using local anesthesia. She tolerated the procedure well according to the documentation. After surgery, Mrs. Johnson was told to use some Ibuprofen if needed for pain, and encouraged to return to using her hand as soon as she could comfortably do so. At her 3-week follow-up appointment with Dr. Azhir, she complained of continued pain and stiffness. Dr. Azhir was concerned at her lack of progress from the previous follow-up visit, and referred her for therapy. In his referral note, the surgeon requested that occupational therapy provide "aggressive treatment to regain mobility, strength, and function" for this client.

That afternoon you hear your name over the department's intercom, notifying you that your new client has arrived. You hear Mrs. Johnson in the waiting room before you see her. When you open the door and ask for Mrs. Johnson, she bustles over to you, saying loudly in a strong southern accent, "Alright now darlin,' let's get this show on the road!" As soon as you seat her in a chair in the treatment room and begin to introduce yourself, she holds her right hand out. "Just look at this! It's not right. Can you fix it?" You immediately notice that the third digit of her hand, along with the palm below the small healing incision is edematous. You can see that the stitches have been removed and the edges of the incision are well approximated.

You begin by asking Ms. Johnson how she typically uses her hands, encouraging her to describe her usual routine. She tells you that she does all the cooking, cleaning, and laundry for her mother and herself, and has found it very inconvenient to have to "rest her hand all the time" since her surgery. She explains that she has had to arrange for an aid to help her and her mother out at home while she recovers from the procedure.

She describes the home where she and her mother live as an older two-story home with a small basement. The bedrooms and bath are upstairs with a small half-bath on the first floor, and the laundry in the basement. She and her mother both live on her mother's social security benefits and a small widow's pension, and whatever she makes from secretarial work. In response to your question about leisure interests, Mrs. Johnson tells you that she loves to watch soap operas and she attends Bible study at her church regularly. She expresses concern that if her hand doesn't improve she may have to retire and begin drawing social security herself, even though it will be financially difficult.

Questions as You Begin

Consider these questions as you begin developing this case:

- You are concerned that Mrs. Johnson isn't really trying to get better, perhaps because she doesn't want to return to work, and is enjoying having some help at home. How do you weigh her right to live her life the way she wants, and your responsibility to try to help her get better?
- The physician has asked for aggressive therapy, but you can't imagine that approach working well with this client. How should you proceed?

CASE

3.10

CLIENT: Gerhard Borgman, 56-year-old Swedish American male

CONDITION: Dupuytren's contracture

SETTING: Outpatient rehabilitation clinic

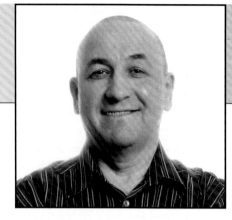

You work in a small rural rehabilitation clinic that is affiliated with the local nonprofit community hospital. As an occupational therapy generalist, you see a wide variety of diagnoses. The local orthopedic surgeon referred a new client to you following surgery to correct a Dupuytren's contracture of his right hand. You were not familiar with the condition and did some research before your new client came in for his evaluation.

You learn that Dupuytren's contracture is a hand deformity where thickened tissue forms bands under the skin of the palm, called palmar fibromatosis, pulling one or more of the fingers into a flexion contracture. It occurs most often in men over the age of 40 and of northern European descent. There is a known genetic link. Other risk factors you note are diabetes and alcoholism, although the association to either condition is not clear.

In reviewing the demographic information in the medical records on this individual, he appears to fit the profile of this condition quite well. You learn that Mr. Borgman is 56 years old and a first-generation Swedish American. His insurance is through one of the large health maintenance organizations (HMOs) that are common in your area. There is no mention in his most recent medical history and physical of diabetes, but you do notice that there is a note about reduced liver function, which could be related to alcohol use. He also has asthma for which he takes Albuteral. Mr. Borgman has no allergies other than seasonal allergies. He works at the local auto body plant as a quality engineer, but has been placed off work by the surgeon for 6 weeks after the surgery. He lives with his wife and has one grown son in college. The personal history section also notes that the client reports he smokes one pack of cigarettes per day and is a "social" drinker.

You scan some scholarly articles on the condition and find that splinting as treatment is controversial, with little evidence to support its use. You also note that recurrence of the condition is common. On the surgeon's referral form, you see that the client's status is 10 days after limited fasciectomy using a common zig-zag incision. The stitches were removed today and Mr. Borgman was to start therapy immediately with the goal to prevent joint stiffness and optimize hand mobility and function. After surgery he was given a prescription for Oxycodone for pain.

Mr. Borgman arrives a few minutes late for his evaluation, apologizing for his confusion over how to find the clinic. You observe that he is a large, muscular man with a booming voice. A small woman accompanies him and sits quietly next to him. He is quite assertive with the secretary, demanding to have all future appointments first thing in the morning. When you introduce yourself, he comments that you don't look old enough to be a very experienced therapist. You assure him that even though his case is rather unique, you have worked closely with his surgeon on many patients over the past several years. You also tell him that you will be happy to give him the earliest appointment you have available, encouraging him to book in advance so he will get a time that he is happy with.

Satisfied, Mr. Borgman follows you back to your evaluation area. You tell him, "Before I unwrap your hand, I need some information. I need to know how you normally use your hand, and what we need to work on first." He seems surprised, and asks why you don't just start fixing his hand. You explain to him that everyone is different, every hand is different. And you have to get things working again as a team. "Are you a welder, a violinist or a bank manager?" Mr. Borgman smiles, "If you could make me a bank manager that would be great!" You start removing his bandage, and he starts telling you about his typical daily routine. You notice that he smells of alcohol and cigarettes. You are glad you read about the surgery beforehand so that you were prepared for the large jagged incision in the palm of Mr. Borgman's right hand. He confirms that he is right-hand dominant. He tells you that the third and fourth fingers of his right hand had been drawn down toward his palm, and could not be straightened, even by pulling on them.

You learn that Mr. Borgman does a lot of writing during the day, as well as operating some machinery, handling moderately heavy tools and equipment, and does some computer work. He rarely does any heavy lifting. He has an assistant at work that he can delegate many of the tasks to. When asked what he likes to do in his free time, he laughs and says, "Hang out with the guys and drink a few brews!" He also adds that he enjoys fishing and hunting.

Questions as You Begin

Consider these questions as you begin developing this case:

- You are concerned that his smoking may slow down the healing process after his surgery. Should you mention this to him?
- Should you mention that alcoholism is a likely contributing factor, and the condition can reoccur?
- If you don't share this, are you denying him the right to possibly make some lifestyle changes?
- You didn't find a specific protocol on rehabilitation of this condition in your research. And you are a little intimidated by the large incision covering most of his palm. How do you know how far to have him move his digits at first?

CASE

3.11

CLIENT:	John Young, 58-year-old Korean American male
CONDITION:	Low back pain (herniation between L5 and S1)
SETTING:	Private outpatient rehabilitation clinic

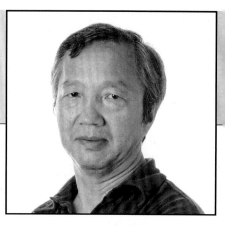

You work in a privately owned rehabilitation clinic in the outskirts of a large city. The clinic is located in a busy plaza, and is next to a fitness center. There are five physical therapists, two physical therapy assistants, yourself, and one other occupational therapist. It is a fast-paced clinic with a very collaborative group of employees.

Today, you review your schedule first thing in the morning and notice that you are scheduled to see a new client named John Young right after lunch. The referral gives a diagnosis of a herniated disc. On the admission paperwork the referring physician has written, "Occupational Therapy to help patient learn how to live with chronic low back pain–patient does not want surgery at this time." You note the following demographic information from the front sheet in the chart: The client is 58 years old, and works as an accountant. He is a Korean American and speaks both Korean and English, and lists Buddhist as his religion. His wife Lea Young is listed as his emergency contact. He has private insurance through his employer. A recent history and physical are included in the chart and reveal that Mr. Young is diagnosed with a herniated disc between his L5 and S1 vertebrae. His symptoms include pain radiating from his lower back down the posterior of both legs, with the right leg more painful than the left. He is unable to rise up on his toes, and has some loss of sensation on the lateral aspect of both feet. This pain had a sudden onset when Mr. Young was doing some gardening outside of his row house in the city. Other information shows that he is moderately obese and has high cholesterol that is managed with medication. He has no allergies, and no other notable health issues. Following the onset of back pain, his overall comfort and function were somewhat improved with physical therapy treatment, epidural cortisone injections, and an oral steroid, methylprednisolone.

The client is now 5 months from the acute onset of his symptoms, and has not made any further improvement in the last 4 weeks. The orthopedic surgeon has recommended a microdiscectomy, but Mr. Young has declined to have the surgery. He wants to return to work and try to manage the symptoms in hopes that his health will continue to improve with more time. Mr. Young is currently having difficulty dressing and bathing, increased pain if he drives for more than half an hour, and cannot do his usual home maintenance activities such as taking out the trash and yard work due to pain with lifting and bending.

Additional personal information gleaned from the chart mentions that Mr. Young changed his name from Geonwoo Jun-young to John Young when he immigrated to the United States as a young man. He lives with his wife Lea of 25 years and he has three daughters, the youngest of whom is in college. His oldest daughter and his grandson live with him and his wife. Mr. Young's interests include traveling with his family to see different parts of the country and reading several newspapers a day to keep up on current events. He dreams of retiring at age 60 and learning to sail. Now he is fearful of re-injuring his back if he does not move carefully enough, and expresses anxiety about his ability to return to work and resume an active lifestyle.

After lunch Mr. Young is brought back to your treatment area. He is wearing a somewhat rumpled red shirt and walks carefully with a slight forward bend at the waist. He looks down watching the ground, and when he is introduced he gives a small bow with his head. You welcome him, nodding your head in return and inviting him to sit in the chair.

Questions as You Begin

Consider these questions as you begin developing this case:

- You are not sure how "traditional" Mr. Young is in his practice of his original cultural traditions. From his use of a bowed head in greeting, you suspect that he may still practice some of them. How can you learn about any cultural traditions that may affect how you work with him?
- You don't feel that you have much training in treating people with low back pain. Even though the primary treatment for this condition has been done by a physical therapist over the past several months, you need to be aware of what the recommendations and precautions are so you can incorporate them into your work with him. How can you get up to speed on this?

Neurologic Cases

Traumatic Neurologic Conditions

In this chapter, you will encounter some of the most common and yet most devastating traumatic injuries that we as therapists treat. In the clinic, I am seeing cerebral vascular accidents with younger and younger clients. The devastation, not just to the client but to the entire family, is far-reaching. To suddenly have your role as wage earner and productive community member disrupted and active leisure pursuits temporarily, if not permanently, impaired would have a profound effect on anyone. Our role is to work with these individuals not only to recover as much function as possible but also to compensate for permanent deficits, and, perhaps most importantly, to help them redefine who they are, what their life goals are, and how they want to engage in valued occupations. Our Therapeutic Use of Self, along with our interactive reasoning skills, is often the key to success, as we develop therapeutic relationships that allow individuals to come to terms with the many changes in their lives.

Occupational therapists will often first see a patient with a traumatic neurologic injury in an intensive care unit or a trauma center. Once medically stable, the client will likely be moved into a more general medical unit that can handle neurologic disorders. When no longer in need of acute services, the client will be assessed to see if they can medically and psychologically tolerate an inpatient rehabilitation facility. Clients with more serious injuries such as traumatic brain injury have been found to have greater improvement if they can participate in inpatient rehabilitation.[1] Acute and postacute treatment may include physical, occupational, and speech therapies and other rehabilitative interventions "…of sufficient scope, timing, intensity and duration [to] restore maximum levels of function and reduce long-term disability and pain, rather than merely accommodating for disability through durable medical equipment or medication.[2]" Outpatient services may follow inpatient rehabilitation with ongoing treatment of clients with traumatic neurologic injuries once they transition back into a community setting. Some students find it intimidating or emotionally stressful to work with these clients and their families soon after the traumatic event. However, those who find they love working with clients suffering from traumatic neurologic conditions will often say that they are humbled and inspired by their work.

CASE 4.1

CLIENT: Kendall Murdock, 42-year-old African American male

CONDITION: Acquired brain injury

SETTING: Hospital inpatient critical care unit; inpatient rehabilitation facility

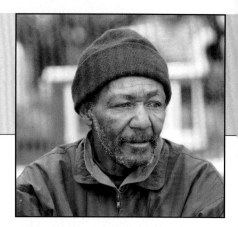

Initial Setting

You work in the rehabilitation department of a large regional medical center. You are assigned to the critical care unit, along with a team of physical, occupational, and speech therapists, respiratory therapists, social workers, dietitians, and critical care nurses. Your schedule is flexible depending on what clients are in the unit, what their conditions are, and how stable they are. This morning you attended the morning report at the 7:00 AM shift change and heard that there was a homeless African American man admitted last night with an acquired brain injury. Nursing noted that he was brought to the emergency department by ambulance after having been assaulted. A friend accompanied him to the hospital and told the staff that the man's name was Kendall Murdock and that both of them were homeless and lived under an overpass. Mr. Murdock was poorly nourished, hypothermic, and had unstable vitals and poor respiratory status when he arrived. A head computed tomography (CT) scan and X-rays revealed a brain injury and a fractured clavicle. The patient was placed on a ventilator to support his respirations and given intravenous fluids, Decadron to reduce swelling in the brain, and Dopamine to control his blood pressure.

A social worker had interviewed the patient's friend and obtained the following additional information: Kendall Murdock was a 42-year-old American veteran who had been homeless since shortly after he left military service 5 years ago with an honorable discharge. He had been divorced while still in the military, and his friend was not aware of any children. His mother was not alive, and his father was in a nursing home in another state. The patient's friend gave his name as Neil, and he claimed that they had both been assaulted by some teenaged boys in a pickup truck with baseball bats. He did not want to file a report with the police, and declined to be treated or give his last name. He was given a bandage for a small cut above his eye before he left. Neil was referred to a shelter, but left the emergency department stating that he was going to return to the overpass to look out for his and Kendall's possessions. He mentioned in passing that Kendall liked animals and used to have a dog that stayed with him. There was no insurance listed for Kendall, although his friend said that he occasionally had hitchhiked to a Veterans' Affairs (VA) hospital in the next town if he needed medical care.

The nurse noted that his vital signs were more stable this morning, and the respiratory therapist reported that they were making progress in weaning Mr. Murdock off the ventilator. The attending physician confirmed the improvement and stated that the patient was beginning to respond to painful stimuli. Physical and occupational therapy were encouraged to see the patient during the day shift to begin therapy to the degree that the patient could tolerate it. After reviewing the blood work that had been ordered, the physician stated he wanted to meet with the dietitian, pharmacist, and nurse on the case to discuss the patient's nutritional and metabolic needs. The physician stated that if Mr. Murdock remained stable for 24 hours, he would be moved out onto the medical floor. The social worker suggested that he would contact the local VA hospital to see if Mr. Murdock should be transferred for care at the VA hospital, or if they can provide rehabilitation if needed after he is medically stable.

By early afternoon you go up to the unit to see how the new patient is doing. Nursing reports that he is off the ventilator now and trying to talk. His eyes are open and focusing on objects, but he is not able to follow simple directions yet. He has pulled one of his intravenous lines out, and nursing staff were trying to consult with the physician about the need to restrain his arms. You ask if you can see him first to attempt to calm him.

The critical care unit is busy today, with multiple glass-walled rooms encircling the nursing station in the middle. Monitors were making varied noises, and lights were on over several rooms. You find Mr. Murdock's room and see that he is moving restlessly in his bed, holding onto one of the side rails and pulling at his blankets. When you enter, he looks at you briefly without interest and then looks away. At the sound of your voice, he looks again at you, but you are not able to maintain his attention by speaking to him. You notice that his hair is matted with blood or dirt, and his hands have dirt caked under the nails.

Questions as You Begin

Consider these questions as you begin developing this case:

- Mr. Murdock is not on any special infection control precautions. Should you put on gown and gloves to work with him?
- You can't really talk about his home and family, so what can you talk to him about? His life is so different from yours, how can you relate to him?

Transfer to Inpatient Rehabilitation Facility

The Del Ray Veterans Hospital has an inpatient rehabilitation facility designed to provide multiple therapies at high frequency and intensity during the early- to middle-recovery phase after serious traumatic injuries such as spinal cord and brain injuries. You work in the occupational therapy department and have just received a new referral for Kendall Murdock. He is being admitted from a regional medical center following 2 weeks of treatment for an acquired brain injury. You turn to the electronic medical record to read up on the background information before you go to meet him. He will probably just be getting settled in today, and his initial interprofessional team meeting will be held this afternoon to set up his schedule and initial goals. You would like to see Mr. Murdock before the meeting.

The face sheet states he has no permanent address; however, he has health insurance through the Veterans Administration Medical Service Package. The medical history and physical report describe a poorly nourished man of 42 years who has been homeless since he left the military 5 years ago. He suffered a closed brain injury after he was assaulted. Over the course of 2 weeks, his Glasgow Coma Scale[3] increased from a 7 to a 15 and he was responding to simple commands. The physical therapy discharge summary from the medical center where he was first treated records left-sided weakness and an ataxic gait, and recommends one assist for transfers and a standard walker for short distances. Occupational therapy completed a Functional Independence Measure[4] on day 3 of his hospital stay and the patient scored a 40. At discharge when it was repeated, he scored a 55, reflecting the need for supervision and setup for meals, moderate assistance for bathing, and maximal assistance with lower body dressing. There was significant impairment noted in memory and executive function, with some lateral neglect of the left side. By discharge, the patient was able to follow simple directions, and gave one- or two-word responses to simple questions.

After completing your review, you decide to visit Mr. Murdock at around 11:00 AM when you have a break between treatments. When you knock on his door, you find that two nursing staff are just clearing an empty meal tray and taking his vitals. When they are finished, you introduce yourself and ask Mr. Murdock if he was hungry. After a slight pause, he answers, "Yes." When you ask him what his favorite food is, he doesn't respond, and looks out the window.

Questions as You Begin

Consider these questions as you begin developing this case:

- You can't imagine that Mr. Murdock will be released back to the streets to live, especially if he has some residual deficits. What kinds of options are available to him?
- Where he is going to live will affect your goals. Should you introduce him to some kind of group sessions, assuming that he will be going to a group setting for housing?
- Or will this be overwhelming for him if he is used to being a "loner?"

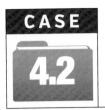

CASE

4.2

CLIENT:	Richard Kunayak, 62-year-old Inuit male
CONDITION:	Left cerebral vascular accident
SETTING:	Hospital inpatient medical unit; transitional care unit

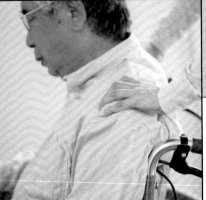

Initial Setting

You work in the inpatient rehabilitation department of Randall County Health Care System, a general hospital in a large city. There are five physical therapists, two occupational therapists, and a speech language pathologist in the department. At times it is frustrating that patients are discharged so quickly, because it seems that you barely get to do much more than evaluate them. You understand that the changes in health care are not going to reverse the trend for quicker discharges. In response to the shortened treatment time, your department has been working hard to meet with physicians and convince them to refer patients to therapy sooner, so you have more time to impact the outcomes before discharge.

Today when you come in and look at the day's treatments, you notice a new referral for a patient who was just moved out of the intensive care unit onto the medical floor. The referral tells you that his name is Richard Kunayak, he is 62 years old, and is in room 107A. His diagnosis is listed as left cerebral vascular accident (CVA). You know that when you complete an evaluation in the morning, you can sometimes fit another treatment session in for the new patient later that same day. You decide to see Mr. Kunayak first today, so you read through his electronic medical record before you go to his room to conduct the initial evaluation. On the patient information sheet, you note that his background is Inuit, and his work is listed as "forestry." He has Worker's Compensation through his employer listed as his insurance. His emergency contact is listed as Sarah Jimmerson.

The personal history notes prepared by the social worker from interviewing Mr. Kunayak and his companion reveal that Mr. Kunayak is divorced and lives with his friend Sarah Jimmerson in a remote cabin in a region that has few services. He is a member of the Inuit tribe from Alaska, and he moved to the state of Washington about 10 years ago with the foresting company he works for. He has no children, and no close family, but he is active in the loose community of Inuit and other Native Americans in the area, according to Ms. Jimmerson. Mr. Kunayak has smoked for many years and uses alcohol occasionally. It was also noted that Mr. Kunayak had been visited in the hospital by his Shaman, an Inuit religious leader.

Under the history of the present illness, you read that Mr. Kunayak was reportedly working in a remote forested area when he became dizzy and lost consciousness. One of the other workmen found him when he did not respond to a radio call, and arranged for Mr. Kunayak to be airlifted to this hospital. The initial computed tomography (CT) scan performed in the emergency department was inconclusive. However, a magnetic resonance imaging (MRI) scan after admission identified the cause of his condition as a clot in his left cerebrum leading to an ischemic cerebral vascular accident. In the medical history and physical report, the attending physician writes that this client has a history of high blood pressure and high cholesterol. It was noted that he has a family history of heart disease and stroke. There is no other significant past medical history listed, and Mr. Kunayak has no known allergies.

Mr. Kunayak was in the intensive care unit for 3 days following his admission, and then transferred to the medical floor. Over the course of his stay in the intensive care unit he became fully responsive, but demonstrated mild expressive aphasia and apraxia. He also had significant right hemiparesis. You note in the medication list that the only medication he has been placed on besides a vitamin is Lisinopril for hypertension, and Spironolactone, a diuretic. The social work note suggests a discharge plan to the hospital's transitional care unit after he has completed his acute care stay. This is a perfect example of what your department is working on. You wish that this patient had been referred when he was still in the ICU, and you wonder how much time you will have to work with him before discharge.

When you knock on his door, a woman's voice says, "Come in." Pushing the door open you see an older man in a hospital gown sitting in the bedside chair next to the nearest bed, and a woman with a coat over her arm is standing by his side. The over-bed table is in front of the patient with a breakfast tray on it, and a lot of food scattered around the edge of the plate. It does not appear that much food has actually been eaten. You introduce yourself and ask the man if he is Mr. Kunayak. He nods his head and tosses a spoon on the tray with his left hand, looking discouraged. The woman introduces herself to you as Sarah Jimmerson and then says, "He's been so frustrated because he feels like he should be able to do more, but he's still getting confused when he tries to do the simplest things!" As you begin chatting with the two of them, you learn from Ms. Jimmerson that Mr. Kunayak loves the outdoors, and when he is not working, he is either hunting or gardening. She whispers quietly to you as she starts to leave, "I would take him home, but I would be afraid to care for him by myself—we live so far from help. I really hope he can get some more of his strength back."

Questions as You Begin

Consider these questions as you begin developing this case:

- Since Sarah Jimmerson is not married to Mr. Kunayak, can you discuss his treatment with her, or include her in treatment?
- What role might his Shaman, or other Native American friends be able to play in his recovery?
- When the note said he lived in a remote area with few services, what does that mean?
- How might you need to adapt your work with him on self-care to prepare him to return to his home?

Transfer to Transitional Care Unit

You work in a busy transitional care unit that is part of Randall County Health Care System. Patients on this unit have a variety of diagnoses and are admitted from the acute care hospital for additional rehabilitation before returning home or moving to a nursing facility. The average length of stay in the transitional care unit is 1 to 3 weeks. Most days you work with your current patients in their rooms for most of the morning to promote independence in morning dressing and bathing routines, then you see new admissions before and after lunch. You typically spend afternoons in the rehabilitation room with your patients who are able to use the different equipment in the clinic as they get stronger and closer to discharge.

On today's schedule, you see that you have a new evaluation with a 62-year-old man named Richard Kunayak who has been diagnosed with a left ischemic CVA. As soon as you are finished with your morning treatments, you sit down to review the electronic medical record on your new patient. Mr. Kunayak had residual right hemi-paresis as a result of the CVA with lower extremity muscle strength measured at 4/5 and upper extremity strength measuring 3/5 as of yesterday when he was discharged from acute care and transferred to the transitional care unit. At discharge he had a weak grasp in his right, dominant hand. In addition, you see that his other symptoms are mild aphasia and apraxia. By the end of his 8-day acute care stay, Mr. Kunayak was beginning to put more words together to form simple sentences, but was still strug-gling with mild apraxia that affected both dressing and self-feeding goals. He was also noted to have a low frustration tolerance. The occupational therapy discharge summary stated that with setup and assistance with fastenings he was able to dress his upper body with a lot of cues, and he needed moderate assistance with lower body dressing. He was able to feed himself and perform simple personal hygiene tasks with setup using adaptive equipment and cueing to use his affected arm and hand. The physical therapy discharge note from acute care states he was able to stand with minimal assistance and was able to roll to his side in bed independently. He was using a stand/pivot transfer at time of discharge to the transitional care unit. Due to weak-ness in his right leg, Mr. Kunayak was using a manual wheelchair with his left hand and foot for mobility for up to 50 ft. You noticed that the discharge planner for your tran-sitional care unit had already started a discharge planning document for this patient. So far, the preliminary discharge plan states simply, "Home with services if possible." You recalled from reading the social work note that he lives with Sarah Jimmerson in a rural area with few services.

You proceed to the client's room and enter at the open door. A nurse is with Mr. Kunayak behind a privacy curtain. You say "Hello" from the doorway, and give your name, stating that you are the occupational therapist and you would like to do an evaluation. The nurse lets you know that she will be finished helping Mr. Kunayak bathe in a few minutes, and you tell them you will return shortly. On your second at-tempt you find Mr. Kunayak alone in his room sitting up in bed. He is wearing a hospital gown, and is looking out the window. He turns when you again give your name, but does not respond. When you ask him how he is today, he just shakes his head. When you ask if he is feeling discouraged, he looks directly at you and says angrily, "Yes! I want to go home. She won't take me home." You sit in the bedside chair and say, "Tell me about home."

Questions as You Begin

Consider these questions as you begin developing this case:

- Mr. Kunayak is so distraught over his desire to go home that you have difficulty get-ting him to focus on anything else. He seems to understand you well, but struggles to express himself. If you help him express his anger and frustration through physi-cally pounding or tearing something, do you think that will make it better or worse?
- He finally gets out enough words for you to understand that he and Sarah had a fight last night about him not wanting to come to the transitional care unit. She has not come to see him yet today and he is afraid she has left him. He begs you to call her for him and shows you her phone number on a piece of paper. He points to the phone next to his bed. Should you help him do this?

CASE

4.3

CLIENT: Janet Lessner, 48-year-old Caucasian
                female

CONDITION: Right cerebrovascular accident

SETTING: Inpatient rehabilitation facility; homecare

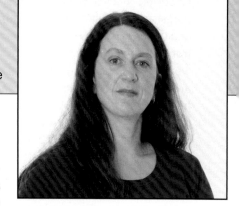

Initial Setting

St. Christopher's is an inpatient rehabilitation facility (IRF) for patients in the early to middle phases
of recovery after a serious traumatic injury. The
majority of patients here have suffered severe central nervous system injuries. These
include traumatic brain injury, spinal cord injury, and cerebral vascular accident. It is
an inpatient program where patients receive therapy and other services for multiple
hours every day. Most of the individuals here have spent several weeks in an acute
care hospital after their injury, receiving services which focused on stabilizing their
medical condition. If patients are unable to tolerate the rigor of treatment at St. Christopher's, they will be transferred instead to either a transitional care unit or skilled
nursing facility for less intensive rehabilitation. St. Christopher's is located in an urban
area, and serves people from a large region because of the specialized care.

     You are a new therapist at St. Christopher's, and are beginning to build a moder-
ate caseload. You are appreciative of the mentoring and support from the other staff
in the department, because many of the cases are very complex. You have also been
encouraged to become familiar with the other services that are provided at the facility,
including physical therapy, speech therapy, rehabilitative nursing, nutrition counselors, medical social workers, and psychologists as well as the attending medical staff.
It is a friendly place to work, and you have developed a real passion for your new job.
You are told that you will be evaluating a new patient today who has suffered a right
cerebral vascular accident (CVA). You start right away to review the information in the
electronic medical record system about your new patient.

     From the demographic data you learn that the referral is for a woman named
Janet Lessner. You are surprised to learn that she is only 48 years old. The next of kin
is listed as her sister. She is Caucasian, and her religious affiliation is listed as Wes-
leyan. Ms. Lessner has private insurance through the local public school system, and
her employment is listed as a teacher. She was transferred to St. Christopher's from a
local medical center, and you can see that there were many tests and treatments done
during her 2-week stay at the hospital. Multiple reports from magnetic resonance imaging (MRI) and computed tomography (CT) scans show that she was diagnosed with
a CVA caused by an intracerebral hemorrhage in the right hemisphere of her brain. You
remember from your training that this type of CVA is typically caused by chronic high
blood pressure. An angiogram of the blood vessels revealed that the damage came
from a rupture of the right middle cerebral artery.

     Next, you turn to the medical history and physical report to gather some more
background information. The chief complaints on admission to the emergency room
were confusion, nausea, difficulty swallowing, paralysis and numbness of the left arm
and leg and drooping of the right side of the face. The history of the present condition
section of the report reveals that the client was teaching her fifth-grade class when

she suddenly became nauseous and dizzy, and called the school nurse for assistance. The school nurse found Ms. Lessner slumped at her desk demonstrating confusion and drooping on the right side of her face. The ambulance was called and she was brought to the emergency department of a local hospital for assessment. In the emergency department, she presented with additional symptoms of difficulty swallowing, and then shortly after admission, loss of consciousness. After intubation and placing her on a ventilator, she quickly underwent a brain scan and it was determined that she was suffering from a brain hemorrhage and cerebral edema was present. Mannitol was administered to reduce the pressure on the brain and minimize secondary cell damage. You note that other than a hysterectomy 3 years ago she had an unremarkable surgical history, but in the medical history section you note that she was previously diagnosed with hypertension.

The personal history section states that Janet Lessner is divorced and lives with her two teenaged daughters, and she has a third daughter in college. She has a long history of smoking at least one package of cigarettes per day, but had recently been trying to quit. She had briefly taken medication for hypertension approximately 2 years ago when she was originally diagnosed, but did not refill her prescription after it ran out. The current medications section in the discharge summary from the hospital lists Hydrochlorothiazide, and a Nicotine patch.

The hospital social work note states that Ms. Lessner owns a three-bedroom, two-storey home in a small town on the outskirts of the city. She went through a contentious divorce 10 years ago with a drawn-out legal battle over custody of her daughters. Her parents live nearby and were caring for the two younger daughters during Ms. Lessner's hospitalization following the CVA. She did not want her ex-husband to know of her hospitalization. Ms. Lessner was concerned about her job, and had financial concerns if she was not able to return to work. She has excellent insurance coverage through the school's health maintenance organization.

On the discharge summary, you note from nursing that the client was cooperative with care, and her confusion had cleared over the course of her stay; however, she continued to have a labile affect with frequent crying spells. She worked with a speech therapist in the hospital and had shown progress with improved swallowing and no longer demonstrated facial drooping on the right, but still has some dysarthria. The occupational therapist at the hospital noted in the discharge plan that Ms. Lessner scored 4 out of 5 for strength of her left shoulder muscles through manual muscle testing, and 3 out of 5 for strength in her left forearm and wrist. Sensory in left upper extremity had improved during her acute care hospital stay, with only a slight impairment remaining with a sharp/dull sensory test. She still had only minimal use of her left hand with only trace contractions and no functional grasp. Moderate visual neglect on the left was also noted. The occupational therapy services at the hospital focused primarily on beginning to address motor, sensory, and perceptual deficits. At the time of discharge she was noted to be independent with setup and adaptive equipment for eating and bathing her upper body. No mention was made about dressing or toileting. Physical therapy notes indicate that at time of discharge from acute care she was transferring independently, ambulating short distances with contact guard and a platform walker, and operating a wheelchair with her strong left arm and both feet for longer distances. The intake form for your facility does not give any additional information other than the plan to discharge home with services when goals are met.

You decide to meet your new patient in her room, and accompany her to the clinic for the initial occupational therapy evaluation. You knock on her door and hear her say, "Come in." You find Janet Lessner in bed, with the room darkened. She is dressed in a nightgown and has a bathrobe nearby. After introducing yourself, you tell her that you would like her to come down to the clinic so that you can evaluate her. She sighs, and then uses her right arm to pull against the side rail to sit up. She takes her time standing and sliding her feet into slippers, putting her robe on over her affected arm first. She asks you to help her tie her sash on the robe. You notice that as she is getting out of bed she leaves her left arm hanging at her side. She sits in the wheelchair in her room and asks you if you want her to wheel the chair herself, or if you are going to push her. You respond that you have heard she is doing well with getting around on her own and you would like to see her do it. You note that her left arm is trapped between her left thigh and the side of the armrest in her chair, but she doesn't seem to notice. When you mention it, she roughly pulls her arm up onto her lap. As you follow her through the door of her room, the left wheel of the wheelchair scrapes the doorway.

You walk with her to the clinic and ask her about her family, and what they like to do in their free time. She says she loves to take her daughters shopping, and sometimes they play board games. She also mentions that she has a small vegetable garden. You are able to understand her quite well in spite of some slurred speech. Before you get to the clinic with her, Mrs. Lessner begins to cry. When you ask her what's wrong, she just shakes her head and keeps going.

Questions as You Begin

Consider these questions as you begin developing this case:

- When she starts crying, is it best if you just ignore it and keep going as though it wasn't happening, or stop and ask Mrs. Lessner about what she is feeling?
- Mrs. Lessner has been placed on a nicotine patch to help her stop smoking. This is probably difficult for her, and may be adding to her stress. Should you talk with her about this to see if there are any coping mechanisms you could help her with, or should you just focus on helping her regain function?

Transfer to Homecare

Your homecare agency covers the eastern side of a large city, and the surrounding suburbs. Today you are seeing a new referral at the end of the day. Over your lunch hour you find a quiet bench in a park and you pull out your company laptop to do some paperwork. After filing notes from the morning's visits, you open the file for your new patient, Janet Lessner. The admission file tells you that this is a middle-aged woman, 48 years old, who has just been discharged home from an inpatient rehabilitation unit. She suffered a hemorrhagic cerebral vascular accident 10 weeks ago, and has spent the last 4 weeks undergoing strenuous rehabilitation for her residual deficits. You turn to the discharge summary to get a better understanding of what her current challenges are.

According to the nursing discharge note from the rehabilitation facility, Ms. Lessner was self-administering her medications consistently with supervision by time of discharge. She was still displaying some labile affect, but this had lessened slowly since admission. Her blood pressure and other vitals were stable. Her medications upon discharge home were Hydrochlorothiazide and a nicotine patch. Although she had started an antidepressant for the first several weeks in the rehabilitation center, she did not tolerate it well and it was discontinued a week before discharge and was not renewed. The social work discharge summary stated that the patient would like to return to work as soon as she is able to, but that she needs to talk to her employer about accommodations. Her endurance was not sufficient to teach all day, and she felt it would be helpful if she could move her room to the first floor, and closer to the teacher's lounge/bathroom. A raised toilet seat and wheeled walker had been ordered from a durable medical equipment supplier to be delivered to her home. Her two teen-aged daughters were going to be home with her, and would be able to provide simple meals and assist with driving when they were not at school.

The physical therapy summary indicated that her balance and strength had im-proved and she was now ambulating up to 200 ft three times per day using a rolling walker. Although she occasionally used a standard wheelchair for longer distances when she was tired, the physical therapist was only recommending a rolling walker for discharge. The strength of her left lower extremity was given as 4/5 using manual muscle testing. Her balance was fair, but she was still demonstrating some left-sided neglect when walking, resulting in veering to the left side of the hall, and not consis-tently noticing objects on her left. Her home had two steps and a railing to enter, and a physical therapist had been working with her on this skill. At this time, she continued to need minimal to moderate assistance to safely ascend and descend two steps. This assistance would be provided by family, and it was recommended that therapy be con-tinued at home to increase her level of independence with this skill. Speech therapy had discharged Ms. Lessner from treatment, but mentioned that organizational skills and executive-level reasoning were still inconsistent, and some assistance might be needed for such things as creating shopping lists and bill-paying.

The occupational therapy discharge note stated that Janet Lessner was able to dress herself using a dressing stick and sock aid, as well as a button hook and zipper pull for fastenings. The therapist recommended a long shower bench with legs inside and outside of the tub to eliminate the need to step into the tub at home. A handheld shower and safety rails were also recommended for safety and independence during showering. These items are supposed to be delivered to the patient's home. She had begun working on meal preparation and was able to make sandwiches and microwave dishes, but still needed cueing for safety when using a stove or oven, and assistance carrying heavy items in the kitchen. Discharge recommendations from occupational therapy included supervision and standby assistance for showering, and dress-ing should be done while sitting to avoid falls. Additional home therapy was recom-mended to continue working toward independence in activities of daily living (ADLs) and the instrumental activities of daily living (IADLs) the patient was most concerned with through restorative and compensatory approaches.

You are pleased with the amount of information you have to inform your assess-ment and treatment planning. At 3:00 PM you ring the front doorbell at the Lessner home. It takes a long time for Janet Lessner to answer the door, and she looks tired and somewhat unkempt when she finally is able to open it. You introduce yourself, and she invites you in, leading the way to the living room. The house is cluttered, with stacks of magazines and papers piled on most of the flat surfaces you can see. Ms. Lessner takes a seat in a comfortable lounge chair with a cluttered end table next to it. When you ask her to tell you how things have been since she got home 3 days ago, she be-gins to cry. "I'm overwhelmed," she tells you, "I didn't think everything would be this hard." After talking with her you discover that some of the adaptive equipment had not been delivered, and no one was home with Mrs. Lessner.

Questions as You Begin

Consider these questions as you begin developing this case:
- If you feel she is not safe alone at home right now, what should you do before you leave at the end of your first session?
- Whose responsibility is it if some of the adaptive equipment are not delivered?
- When you ask her what is the most frustrating thing for her since she got home she says, "The bills!" She has found a pile of unpaid bills from the past 6 weeks since her hospitalization. Is there anything you can do to help her with this? Should you?
- Since money management does not represent an imminent danger to her safety, are there other issues you should address first?

CASE		
4.4	**CLIENT:**	Eduardo Rodriguez, 39-year-old Hispanic male
	CONDITION:	Radial nerve injury
	SETTING:	Physician-owned outpatient rehabilitation clinic

You work in a busy outpatient rehabilitation clinic owned by an orthopedist. It is located next to a general hospital in a suburban area and treats a variety of patients with conditions that are mostly neurologic or musculoskeletal. You also receive referrals from specialists who practice in the mid-sized city nearby. The clinic has a mixture of physical, occupational, and speech therapists as well as certified occupational and physical therapy assistants. Therapists and assistants are paired up and carry a caseload together. In this way clients know that they will always see "their" therapist or assistant when they come in. When you sit down with Peter, your assistant, to go over the day's schedule you see that you have a new evaluation. The diagnosis for your new client is right radial nerve injury, status postrepair. The referral is from Dr. Lee, a neurologist in the city with whom you are familiar.

You know that nerve injuries can be complex, and decide you will need more information before you see the client this afternoon. You ask the secretary if she would call Dr. Lee's office and ask to have any background information on this client faxed to you as soon as possible so that you can review it prior to the client's arrival. When you break for lunch, you are pleased to find a large packet of information on Mr. Rodriguez.

On the front sheet you see that Eduardo Rodriguez is 39 years old. His employment is listed as "seasonal farm worker." His insurance is listed as Worker's Compensation through the local farm where he is employed. You note that Mr. Rodriguez' primary language is Spanish, and his religious affiliation is listed as Catholic. Next of kin is Maria Rodriguez, his wife.

Next, you look for the medical history and physical report and carefully study the same for additional background information. The first section is under the title "Social History." You read that Eduardo Rodriguez was born in central Mexico and educated through the eighth grade. He then moved with his family to Arizona and went into the fields to work in order to help support his family. His parents moved the family frequently in order to get work wherever crops were being harvested in the southwest. He married Maria when he was 18, and continued in this line of work. Mr. Rodriguez and his wife have four children between the ages of 5 and 16. They have been living in a trailer that serves as fieldworker housing on the farm. He does not have a car, and relies on his employer for transportation. Spanish is his primary language and it is noted that he speaks little English.

Family history shows only that his mother died at age 50 in a motor vehicle accident, and his father died from a myocardial infarction at age 54. There is no information provided about siblings or grandparents. The chief complaint on admission is listed as "decreased ability to move and feel with right arm and hand." The history of the present illness/condition in the medical record describes what led to the referral for therapy. It seems that Mr. Rodriguez was using a tool in the field that required him to lean his right axilla against the metal frame. After a 10-hour day in the field, he complained of weakness and numbness in his right arm. The next morning, he attempted to use the tool again, but was unable to due to worsening weakness and numbness in his right arm and hand. He was brought to the emergency room and then referred to the neurologist. In the assessment and plan, Mr. Rodriguez was diagnosed with radial nerve palsy, taken off work, and put on Gabapentin (Neurontin) for nerve pain and Ambien to help him sleep. He was referred to therapy for strengthening and to promote return of function of his right upper extremity.

The review of systems from the physician shows a well-nourished male with normal vital signs and no remarkable past medical history except for asthma. Significant weakness was noted in his right triceps, wrist, and finger extensors, and numbness was noted down the back of his right arm and on the sides and back of his right thumb, index, and middle fingers. His right grasp was weak, but he was able to make a full composite fist. He could only partially extend his fingers and right wrist after making a fist.

Mr. Rodriguez came to the clinic a few minutes late. He wore blue jeans and a clean blue work shirt, and he was carrying a baseball cap. The department secretary had arranged for an interpreter to assist Mr. Rodriguez during the session. After he was done filling out paperwork, you greet both the client and John, the interpreter and introduce yourself. You accompany them both to your treatment area and begin by asking Mr. Rodriguez what he would like to be called. With the help of the interpreter he encourages you to call him "Eddy." You notice that Eddy is holding and rubbing his right arm, keeping it adducted and internally rotated, with his right forearm across his abdomen. You ask him about pain, pulling out a pain rating scale with faces on it. He points to the face that has tears on it, then looks at John and points instead to the one just before it, where there is a grimacing face, but no tears. After pointing, he rubs his entire right arm and speaks to the older man in Spanish. John tells you that Eddy says the pain is very bad in his entire right arm, making it impossible for him to sleep, eat, or do anything. You nod your head in understanding.

You ask him to tell you more about his work, and other things he does with his hands. With John's help translating, you learn that Eddy works in the field harvesting vegetables for sometimes 10 to 12 hours a day. His two older children and wife also work on the farm. In the evenings he likes to play dominoes and carve wood figures for the small children on the farm. His biggest concern he says is being able to lift and carry for his job. He says in Spanish, "I am a father. I am a husband. I must take care of my family. I must return to my work as soon as I can."

Questions as You Begin

Consider these questions as you begin developing this case:

- Mr. Rodriguez is very concerned about returning to work. He tells you if the pain will subside, he thinks the work will help him get his strength back, so he probably won't need therapy once the pain stops. What should you say to this?
- You feel that using the interpreter interferes with your ability to develop a therapeutic relationship with your client. How can you ensure good communication but still develop a positive relationship?

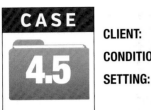

CASE

4.5

CLIENT: Miyu Tanaka, 37-year-old Asian female

CONDITION: Spinal cord injury

SETTING: Inpatient rehabilitation facility; For-profit homecare agency

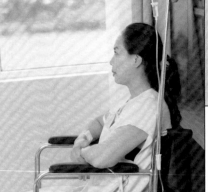

Initial Setting

You work in an inpatient rehabilitation facility (IRF) that is part of a large regional medical center in a mid-sized city. Patients in the IRF have typically suffered serious traumatic injuries such as amputation, traumatic brain injury, spinal cord injury, or cerebral vascular accident. This inpatient unit admits patients from acute-care hospitals for intensive rehabilitation prior to returning home. Most of the individuals here have spent several weeks in an acute care hospital after their injury, receiving services to stabilize their medical conditions. After they have completed their rehabilitation, most clients will be discharged home or to a skilled nursing facility. Therapy for most patients is divided into morning and afternoon sessions. A typical schedule would be to have an hour of occupational therapy (OT) in the morning followed by a half hour of physical therapy (PT), then appointments with social workers, rehabilitation nurses, dietary personnel, or psychologists, and then more therapy in the afternoon–perhaps another half hour of OT and an hour of PT.

This morning, you review your schedule and notice that you will have a new patient to evaluate at 10:00 AM. You find the referral form and see that the new patient is Miyu Tanaka, a 37-year-old female who suffered a complete spinal cord injury (SCI) at the level of the seventh cervical vertebrae (C7) 3 weeks ago. She was moved to the IRF yesterday after a week in ICU and then two more weeks on an acute care medical floor of a local hospital. You turn to the electronic medical record for more information. The demographic information indicates that the patient is Japanese American, with both Japanese and English listed as her primary language. Under occupation it indicates she is a homemaker. Mrs. Tanaka is married and her husband Michael is a financial analyst. The religious affiliation indicated in the medical record for the patient is Buddhist. She has private insurance through her husband's employer.

The medical history and physical report indicate under history of present illness that the patient was pushed onto the tracks in the subway, suffering a spinal fracture in the fall. She lives with her husband and son in an apartment in a nearby town. She does not smoke or drink alcohol. The patient does not work outside of the home. She immigrated to the United States from Japan as a teenager. Mrs. Tanaka developed mild pneumonia while in the hospital, which is resolving. She is being discharged on Avelox to address the lung infection and Lyrica for neuropathic pain.

The discharge nursing note states that the incision from the tracheotomy used when she was first admitted is healing well. There are no other skin integrity problems, and her pain is under good control with current medications. Nursing also notes that the patient is not comfortable with males providing personal care.

The social work assessment note indicates that the client and her family live in a two-bedroom apartment in the city. The note indicates that the couple has a son, 10 years old, named John. According to Mr. Tanaka, John is being cared for by his parents until Mrs. Tanaka returns home. Attempts to discuss long-term management of

Mrs. Tanaka's care have so far not progressed, with both the client and her husband not responding to questions regarding potential homecare services or equipment that would be needed. The discharge plan in the chart at this time is home with services, but the social work note indicates that nursing home placement may need to be explored depending on progress.

The hospital discharge note states that Mrs. Tanaka has made some progress in bed mobility, improving from maximum assistance to moderate assistance needed. She has only been out of bed for brief periods using a mechanical lift. The occupational therapist has been able to engage her in upper body bathing with adaptive equipment such as a bath mitt, and moderate assistance. She is listed as having an interest in sewing and window gardening.

When you enter her room on the IRF unit to introduce yourself, there is a policeman present interviewing the client and her husband about the assault. Mrs. Tanaka seems distressed and tearful, and her husband is holding her hand. Mr. Tanaka is doing most of the talking, and the policeman is trying to get Mrs. Tanaka to answer directly. Mrs. Tanaka is keeping her head down and will not look at the policeman. You notice that she is moving her upper arms including bending her elbow to rub her nose with the back of her wrist. After introducing yourself and asking if you should come back later, the policeman says he is finished. Both the patient and her husband look relieved, and seem to relax after he leaves. You smile at both of them and state that you are sorry to come at a stressful time. Mr. Tanaka encourages you to sit in the remaining chair.

Questions as You Begin

Consider these questions as you begin developing this case:

- The nursing staff and social worker have expressed frustration that Mrs. Tanaka does not try to use her remaining abilities to help herself. They have tried to talk with her about this, but she rarely will discuss anything about her condition. When they speak with her alone she says, "I must wait until my husband is here." How will you approach her to establish a therapeutic relationship and gain her trust?
- Can you leverage her spiritual beliefs to motivate her in her recovery?

Transfer to Homecare

The Premier Home Care Agency is a for-profit firm that provides in-home services to clients in multiple small towns and villages that make up the suburbs to the north of a mid-sized city. You have been working for the agency for several years, finding that you enjoy both the flexibility and independence you have in setting your schedule as well as the challenge of helping people in their natural environments. This morning, you will be going to an apartment to evaluate Miyu Tanaka, a 37-year-old woman who recently suffered a complete spinal cord injury at the seventh vertebral level of the spinal cord. You have already read the information available from the referring facility, and are pleased that there was quite a bit of therapy-related information provided for this challenging case.

From the electronic medical record you also learned that she has received 6 weeks of intensive rehabilitation following her hospital stay. She lives with her husband and 10-year-old son in a two-bedroom apartment. It appears from the discharge information that Mrs. Tanaka has been very slow to make progress in therapy. This was felt to be due to a combination of emotional trauma from her assault as well as cultural barriers. Mr. Tanaka only visited in the evenings, and Mrs. Tanaka left decision-making to him. The couple was not willing to consider nursing homecare for Mrs. Tanaka after discharge, but they were also hesitant to have staff from an outside agency come into their home. Mr. Tanaka insisted that the family would provide for her care needs, but he was vague in describing how this would happen.

The physical therapist recommended that Mrs. Tanaka have an electric wheelchair, as she had been mostly unsuccessful in using a manual chair with push knobs on the rims. By discharge she was able to do a slide board transfer with minimal to moderate assistance, and was cooperative with strengthening exercises for her upper extremities. She was able to independently perform pressure relief activities when sitting in the wheelchair. The occupational therapy discharge note reported that Mrs. Tanaka was able to bathe and dress her upper body after setup using adaptive equipment. She needed moderate assistance and a lot of cueing to complete lower body bathing and dressing. She used a plate guard and universal cuff as well as a passive-grip cup for feeding. Toward the end of her rehabilitation stay the occupational therapist had focused on simple meal preparation and developing independent leisure interests. Mrs. Tanaka had engaged in these activities, but frequently stated that her kitchen was different at home, and she didn't know if she would be able to do anything in her kitchen.

You are not sure who will be at the home when you visit, but you did find time since you received the referral 2 days ago to do some work online to find some information about the Japanese culture. When you arrive at the apartment an elderly Asian woman answers the door. She bows her head when you introduce yourself but does not speak, and shows you into a side bedroom. As you follow her you notice the rooms are very clean, and nicely but sparsely furnished. The medium-sized kitchen is open to the combined living/dining room, with a counter to divide it from the common area. There is something cooking on the stove that smells delicious. Mrs. Tanaka is sitting in a bedside chair in a large, neat bedroom. She is wearing a simple house dress and slippers. You notice several plants on a stand in the corner of the room, a writing desk with magazines on it, and a small television, which the older woman turns off as she enters. You say hello and introduce yourself, explaining simply what you do. Mrs. Tanaka asks you to call her Miyu, and welcomes you to her home. When you look back, the older woman has disappeared.

Questions as You Begin

Consider these questions as you begin developing this case:

- Should you ask probing questions about the people who are providing care for her at home? Or just focus on increasing her independence?
- Would it be considered disrespectful to the older woman and her role to work with Miyu in the kitchen?
- How can you use what you learn about the Japanese culture or Buddhism to help you develop a positive therapeutic relationship with Mrs. Tanaka?
- How can this information inform your practice?

Progressive Neurologic Conditions

Many times, persons living with progressive neurologic conditions make incremental accommodations as the disease progresses. But when there is a more sudden change, they may seek out rehabilitation for assistance in either restoring function or otherwise accommodating to the change. Kern and Brown have speculated that individuals with progressive neurologic conditions often report that quality of life is maintained even when health status declines are measureable, and speculate that this is due to disease adaptation.[5] In other words, the person learns to live with the progressive physical symptoms. Engstrom, Norberg, and Nordeson found that people with progressive neurologic disorders who visited rehabilitation clinics more often reported significantly higher quality of life than those who did not.[6] Taken together, these reports would seem to indicate that many of our clients with chronic neurologic conditions have a significant capacity to both adapt incrementally as the disease process progresses, and to benefit from supportive interventions such as occupational therapy. The following cases present four different progressive disorders of the nervous system that are commonly encountered in occupational therapy. Individuals with these conditions will generally be seen in outpatient, homecare or skilled nursing settings, where you will assist them with interventions to support occupational adaptation and improved performance.

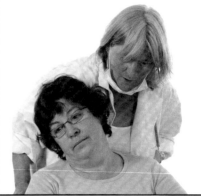

CASE

4.6

CLIENT: Sandra Livingstone, 63-year-old Native American female

CONDITION: Multiple sclerosis

SETTING: Medical model day program; skilled nursing facility

Initial Setting

You have just received a new referral for the medical model day program where you work. The program is part of the Phillips Long Term Care Center that provides a variety of levels of care for individuals with chronic illnesses. The day program is an outpatient program designed for persons living in the community with medical or cognitive problems who require one or more skilled services such as physical or occupational therapy, or skilled nursing care. The clients live at home with family and attend the program 2 to 5 days a week. In addition to skilled services, the program monitors chronic conditions such as diabetes, and provides a hot meal and recreational and social activities. You perform an initial occupational therapy (OT) evaluation on each client and either provide skilled OT services directly, or consult with the program's nursing and activities personnel to assist in developing a plan that will engage the clients in valued occupations and enhance personal performance. Support services are also available to clients in the program from the facility's dietitian and pharmacist as needed.

The new referral is for a woman named Sandra Livingstone who is diagnosed with relapsing-remitting multiple sclerosis (MS). She currently lives outside of this rural, New England town with her daughter and daughter's family. The referral to the program from the patient's primary care physician requests therapy to assist Sandra Livingstone with generalized strengthening and to maintain function so that she can continue to live with her family.

Your review of the medical records for Mrs. Livingstone shows that she is a 63-year-old Native American woman from the Algonquian tribe. She is moderately obese and has been diagnosed with MS since she was 35. She was widowed approximately 10 years ago and lived alone until 2 years ago when it became too difficult for her to care for her home and prepare meals. Since then she has lived with her daughter, son-in-law, and two grandchildren. A home care agency has provided a nurse to give her intravenous medications for her MS once per month, and an aide comes twice a week to help her with showering.

Recently her symptoms have worsened with increasing weakness in her legs and arms, decreased balance, and diminished vision. She now uses a wheelchair even in the home, and gets around using her feet to move the chair. She is usually alone at home for most of the day while her daughter and son-in-law work and her grandchildren are at school. The homecare agency decided to terminate care after nursing notes indicated that the client had a series of falls while she was home alone. Although she didn't suffer any serious injuries, the agency was concerned that she was no longer safe at home alone. The homecare agency recommended that she be admitted to either a full-time day program or a nursing home, so that she was no longer left home alone.

On the discharge summary from the homecare nurse, it says that the client's family hopes that Mrs. Livingstone can attend a day program 5 days per week instead of considering admission to a nursing home. Further information reveals that Mrs. Livingstone transfers independently but sometimes forgets to put her brakes on in her wheelchair, and needs moderate assistance with showering and dressing her lower extremities. When she was discharged from the homecare agency, she was on intravenous Methyl prednisone once per month to slow the progression of her multiple sclerosis, and Bactrim for a UTI. Mrs. Livingstone receives Social Security disability, Medicaid, and healthcare coverage under the Indian Health Service.

When you meet her at the day program evaluation preliminary visit, Mrs. Livingstone is pleasant, and says she is looking forward to coming to the program. She is oriented and easily follows one- and two-step directions, and responds appropriately in conversation. She is especially interested in the rehabilitation aspects of the program so she can get a little stronger and "not be a burden" on her family. She also says she is looking forward to being with people during the day. Mrs. Livingstone's daughter, Lisa, came with her today and is tearful at times as she listens to her mother. Lisa expresses guilt at not being able to stay home to provide care for her mother. When asked about her leisure interests, Mrs. Livingstone says, "Playing with my grandchildren, watching game shows, and baking cookies." Lisa stayed for the entire time with her mother. She expressed some concern later about her mother being a lot more "with it" than some of the participants, and wondered if this was the best place for her mother.

Questions as You Begin

Consider these questions as you begin developing this case:

- How should you respond to the daughter's concerns about her mother being with people who are not as cognitively alert?
- Should you have tried to convince the daughter to let her mother spend some of this first day at the program by herself?

Transfer to Skilled Nursing Facility

You are an occupational therapist working for the residential skilled services unit of the Phillips Long Term Care Center. You have just finished a morning care planning meeting on the unit, and were informed by the head nurse that there was a new resident admitted this morning with a diagnosis of multiple sclerosis (MS). You know the facility's policy is that all initial evaluations must be completed within 24 hours of admission, so you check your schedule as soon as you return to your office. It appears that the best time for you will be late afternoon today, but you realize that the patient might be tired by then. You see the physical therapist at her desk and stop to coordinate with her. You both decide to complete your evaluations on the new resident tomorrow morning–you will ask the nursing staff not to do morning dressing and care with the new resident, so that you can evaluate her during this activity, and the physical therapist will see her after breakfast. Later that day you go up to the nursing unit to look at the medical record for the new resident to gather information for your evaluation.

Sandra Livingstone is a 68-year-old woman who has been attending the facility's medical model day program for the past 5 years. You see on the chart that the resident has Medicare Part A and Part B, Medicaid, and Indian Health Service coverage.

During the past 5 years, she lived with her daughter and daughter's family, but gradually needed more assistance with personal care. It was Mrs. Livingstone's decision to move to the facility, so that she would not be a "burden" on her family. The move seemed to be precipitated by the last grandchild going away to college. Her daughter and son-in-law both work outside of the home. Last year, Mrs. Livingstone's diagnosis was changed from relapsing-remitting type MS to secondary-progressive type. You know that the change in her diagnosis indicates that her symptoms are progressing more steadily.

Discharge notes from the day program indicate that Mrs. Livingstone is a one-person assist for transfers, and she is only able to move her manual wheel chair for very short distances. She is oriented in all spheres, but has begun to have a labile affect and some impairment of executive function. Mrs. Livingstone is very social with the other residents, often looking out for others, especially those residents who are frail or confused. She is incontinent and has alternated between using an indwelling catheter and intermittent catheterization. She has been treated for frequent urinary tract infections. She needs moderate assistance for dressing and bathing, due to low endurance.

The next day you go to Mrs. Livingstone's room at 7:00 AM. She is already awake and waiting for you. When you ask about her usual morning routine she tells you, "I've always been an early riser. I get up before the sun—that's the way I was raised."

Questions as You Begin

Consider these questions as you begin developing this case:

- Mrs. Livingstone has lived with her daughter and grandchildren for quite a few years. How can you help her stay connected to her family on a regular basis?
- She is a member of the Algonquin Tribe. Are there any cultural aspects of this background that you should be aware of as you begin treatment?

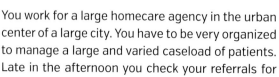

CASE

4.7

CLIENT: Dale Forsythe, 18-year-old Caucasian
                 male
CONDITION: Muscular dystrophy
SETTING: Homecare agency

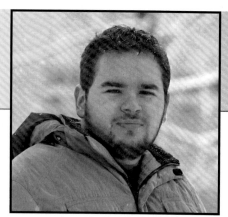

You work for a large homecare agency in the urban center of a large city. You have to be very organized to manage a large and varied caseload of patients. Late in the afternoon you check your referrals for the next day and see that you have a young client to see who has muscular dystrophy (MD). You use the laptop provided by your agency to connect to the Internet and search the database for additional information on your new client.

The referral form states that Dale Forsythe is 18 years old and has Duchenne Muscular Dystrophy (DMD). Next of kin is listed as his father, Dale Forsythe. You note that under employment it lists "student." Religious affiliation was noted as Jewish. He is covered by Supplemental Security Income and Medicaid, which he just received since he turned 18. You switch to the medical history and see that Dale was diagnosed with DMD at the age of 4. Dale has no surgical or other medical conditions listed but you note that he was recently seen at the doctor's office due to an increase in muscle spasms, and the onset of bladder spasms related to his condition. He has moderate scoliosis that has developed slowly over the past 5 years. He has no cardiac problems listed which you are glad to see, knowing that they can be a complication as this condition progresses. Dale uses a manual wheelchair, and at this time is unable to stand or walk independently. His recent decrease in independence and function has prompted the new referral to occupational therapy. He is currently taking Flexeril for muscle spasms and was placed on Ditropan to decrease the bladder spasms.

In the personal history section, you find notes related to his family context. Dale has an older sister and younger brother, neither of whom have the inherited condition. He lives with his parents and siblings in a large row house in an upscale area of the city. His father is an architect and his mother works part time as a music teacher. His older sister is attending a local college. Daniel will graduate from high school at the end of the year with strong grades, and wants to attend a local community college. He is very outgoing and has been actively engaged at school in many extra-curricular activities, participating in the school band and student politics.

You call the phone number listed to make an appointment to complete the initial occupational therapy evaluation tomorrow. Mrs. Forsythe answers the phone. When you introduce yourself and ask to speak with Dale, Mrs. Forsythe asks if she can help you. After explaining that you would like to make an appointment to see Dale, Mrs. Forsythe begins to tell you his schedule. You thank her for the information and ask to speak with Dale in order to "firm up" the appointment. After a brief pause, Mrs. Forsythe leaves the phone and you can hear her talking to her son. When Dale comes on the phone, he speaks clearly and seems self-confident. After agreeing to a time to meet tomorrow and getting directions from Dale you hang up.

The next afternoon, you easily locate Dale's residence from his directions. His mother answers your knock and invites you into the family living room where Dale is sitting in his wheelchair. You see that he is wearing warm-up pants and a football jersey, and has new-looking sneakers on. He smiles easily and puts his hand out in greeting. You ask Dale about the results of his high school's football game last night and he enthusiastically describes their win. His mood darkens, however, when you ask him to tell you about his recent change in symptoms related to the muscular dystrophy. When he hesitates, his mother jumps in, giving you a lot of detailed information about muscle spasm and weakness, some coordination problems as well as difficulty managing his bowel and bladder symptoms. Dale blushes and looks at the floor. After she finishes, you thank her and turn to Dale and say, "Now I'd like to know how you feel about all this—how is it affecting what you want to do with your life?" He leans forward, staring at you intently. "I'm glad you asked me that," he says, "I want to go to college to become a research scientist."

Questions as You Begin

Consider these questions as you begin developing this case:

- Dale's mother appears to be very overprotective. How can you encourage her to support Dale's independence?
- His goal to be a research scientist is probably unrealistic given his progressive condition. Should you talk with him about that?
- Should you get involved with helping establish a bowel and bladder routine, or talk to the nurse about it first?

CLIENT: Darnel Parker, 60-year-old African American male

CONDITION: Parkinson's disease

SETTING: Outpatient rehabilitation clinic

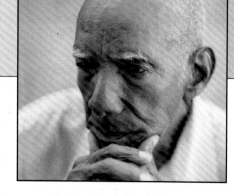

Darnel Parker is a 60-year-old man with a diagnosis of Parkinson's disease. He is a new patient at your outpatient rehabilitation clinic and you will be doing his initial occupational therapy (OT) evaluation. Your clinic is part of a nonprofit community health center in a small town, a suburb of a larger city nearby. You are the only occupational therapist at the center, and you cover the diverse case load with the help of Lisa, an OT assistant. Before Mr. Parker arrives, you review the available information to find out more about him. You are fortunate that Dr. Wilson's office sent over some background information from the medical record.

Included in the information are several key documents: the face sheet with demographic information, the most recent medical history and physical report, and the latest medical progress note. From the face sheet you learn that Mr. Parker is African American, currently married, and lists his religion as Baptist. His health insurance coverage is provided through the Medicaid program. He lives in an apartment building on the edge of the nearby city, about 10 miles from the clinic. The medical history and physical report note the client's chief complaint as "Walking and using hands is getting worse." Under the section titled "History of Present Illness," you see that he has had progressively worsening Parkinson's disease for the past 6 years. He has also smoked two packs of cigarettes a day for many years.

There is no significant surgical history, and the medical history reflects hypertension and occasional depression. Mr. Parker is taking Sinemet to manage his tremors and Norvasc for hypertension in addition to a multivitamin.

In the social history section of the medical history and physical report, you find that he has been married three times, for the past 15 years to his current wife, Sandy. He has children from each of his marriages, with two teenaged children still at home. As his Parkinson's disease has worsened, his wife states he has become more and more dependent on her to leave lunch prepared and manage all of the housework and family finances. They live in an upstairs apartment in an old two-storey house. Sandy works two jobs outside of the home. The client reportedly used to look after the children, but his wife states that since his condition has worsened, he is not helpful and the children are becoming "wild and unsupervised." He used to own his own cab, and still talks as though he is working, when in fact he hasn't been able to work for the past 6 years, since shortly after he was diagnosed with Parkinson's disease. Mr. Parker is left in the house alone for most of the day.

The medical progress note from a recent visit notes that Darnel Parker's pill-rolling tremors and festinating gait have recently worsened. Dr. Wilson feels there is little else she can do to manage his Parkinson's related symptoms with medication adjustments. She notes that the client may no longer be safe to stay at home alone. Dr. Wilson recommends a trial of therapy to see if there are compensatory techniques that may help the client to remain independent and safe at home.

Mr. Parker enters your clinic today with a shuffling narrow-based gait, no arm swing, and demonstrates the typical halting gait as though he is "glued to the floor." His wife is carrying his cane, and when asked she says Darnel tends to just carry it rather than use it. Mrs. Parker hooks her arm through his so she can help him move forward. His speech is in a monotone, and he has a very low volume. His posture is leaned forward in both standing and walking. He has limited facial expression and demonstrates a pill-rolling tremor with his fingers at rest. He stops to sit in a chair halfway across the gym to your work area, saying he needs to rest. Mrs. Parker says she has had to miss work to bring him to the clinic today, and she is concerned about transportation if he needs to come for additional appointments. You pull up a chair near Mr. Parker to talk with him while he rests. He maintains eye contact with you during the conversation, but appears sad and answers with only one- or two-word responses. When you ask him what is the most frustrating part of his day, he answers, "I'm useless." In response to asking him what he likes to do when he is feeling better, he tells you he likes to read the newspaper, play checkers, and go out to the local diner with some "old buddies."

When you ask the couple about entering and leaving the house and transportation, she replies, "It's a fiasco. I had to get a neighbor to help me get him downstairs today." They did confirm that once he is in the apartment, Mr. Parker is able to go into all of the rooms by taking his time and holding onto furniture.

Questions as You Begin

Consider these questions as you begin developing this case:

- You are feeling a lot of pressure with this case, because his wife has to work and says the children are "unreliable" in helping their father, and the doctor is worried that the client is not safe at home anymore. You don't want to be the one to make the decision that he has to go into a nursing home, but if you say he is safe, and then he falls, you will feel responsible. Should you start by having a candid conversation with Mr. Parker and his wife about this decision and what is at stake?
- What are Mr. Parker's rights in this decision?

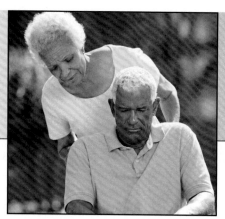

CASE 4.9

CLIENT: Samuel Duncan, 62-year-old African American male

CONDITION: Alzheimer's dementia

SETTING: Medical model day program at a continuing care center; skilled nursing facility with dementia unit

Initial Setting

You have a great job working for a continuing care retirement community that offers multiple levels of services for senior citizens. These levels of care include independent living with access to services, a rest home level where each client or couple has their own room but shared living space and personal care services, a day program, on-site medical offices, outpatient therapy services, and a full-skilled nursing facility. Your occupational therapy position is shared between clients in the skilled nursing facility and the day treatment program. Your role with the day program is mostly consultative with the staff to adapt services to a variety of client needs. Today you have been asked by the day program's director to come to a meeting at the day program to meet Samuel Duncan, a resident from the independent living center. He and his wife have requested to see the program to decide if it would be good for Mr. Duncan to attend. The director tells you that she hopes you will be able to help the staff develop a suitable care plan. You ask her to send you the referral request through the online in-house system, and agree to attend.

You are curious about this request, and complete your other paperwork early enough to gather some background information before leaving for the day program. The facility maintains a proprietary documentation system where personal medical information is protected, but at the same time available to those staff who need it throughout the organization for care purposes. By the time you log into the system, the referral has been entered for you to consult on this client, so you can now access Mr. Duncan's information.

You are surprised to find in the demographic information that Mr. Duncan is only 62 years old, since most of the residents are much older. Couples can live at the center as long as one of them is at least 60, and Mr. and Mrs. Duncan moved in 2 years ago. In the medical data report, you see that in addition to mild rheumatoid arthritis, Samuel Duncan has sickle cell anemia and early-onset Alzheimer's disease. He is African American and lists his religious affiliation as Methodist. The couple has long-term-care insurance that pays for any long-term-care medical expenses. In the personal history, you see that he and his wife Margaret have raised two children who live nearby. He was a postman until taking early retirement at age 56 after being diagnosed with Alzheimer's disease.

The medical history report describes a man of short stature and low weight, who has chronic joint pain related to sickle cell anemia. Due to damage to his spleen from this disorder, he is also plagued with frequent infections. The report clarifies that Mr. Duncan first noticed memory problems when he was unable to learn a new delivery route at work, shortly before his retirement. Subsequent comprehensive testing resulted in a diagnosis of early-onset Alzheimer's disease, of the common type. Over the course of the next 6 years he became increasingly impaired, requiring someone to direct him for common routines, and having to give up driving and yard work. At this time his wife takes care of all of their finances and does all of the cooking and other housework. Mr. Duncan still enjoys playing with his grandchildren, watching the news, and chatting with neighbors. He uses a wheelchair for longer distances because he tires easily, and has started falling when he is tired. He is currently taking Aricept for his dementia, and Hydroxyurea for sickle cell anemia.

You arrive at the cheerful dayroom that is used by the program and see an African American man in a wheelchair who appears much older than 62 years, with a woman sitting next to him holding his hand. You recognize the others in the room as the director, the program's nurse, and the activities assistant. The director introduces you to Mr. and Mrs. Samuel Duncan. She tells you that the couple lives in the independent housing area, but they are here today to discuss Mr. Duncan possibly attending the social-model day program.

You express your pleasure in meeting them both and ask if they have already had a chance to tour the facility and talk with the staff. Mrs. Duncan confirms that they have, and comments that she thinks it might be just what they need. You ask her to tell you how the program would help them both. She starts by turning to her husband and saying, "Samuel, you get bored sometimes during the day since you don't have a yard to care for. Do you think you would enjoy coming here? It would help me too, because I could get my hair done while you're here." Mr. Duncan pats her hand and answers, "I suppose." You ask about their current routine, and are not surprised to find that the couple has developed a variety of coping mechanisms to compensate for Mr. Duncan's increasing memory impairment. You notice that he seems only partly aware of his deficit. Then Mrs. Duncan turns away from her husband and quietly comments to you, "I know he will need the nursing home someday, but I'm hoping with the help of the day program that I will be able to keep him at home as long as possible."

Questions as You Begin

Consider these questions as you begin developing this case:

- At 62 years old, you realize that Mr. Duncan is much younger than the other clients in the program. He would also be the only African American and one of only two men in the program. How could the program be adjusted so that it would be relevant and interesting for Mr. Duncan?
- What aspects of the program are most beneficial for Mrs. Duncan?
- Many individuals with Alzheimer's dementia do not adjust well to change. If Mr. Duncan is to begin coming to the program, how can they make the change easier for him?

Transfer to Skilled Nursing Facility—Dementia Unit

You work at a continuing care retirement community with the dementia care unit. Most of the clients on this 25-bed unit are in the middle to advanced stages of dementia. The ages of your clients range from the mid-50s up to the mid-90s. The unit is designed specifically for residents who need specialized care due to a combination of confusion, overall cognitive decline, and maladaptive behaviors. Many of the residents are still quite mobile, ambulating independently or with assistive devices. The clients are challenging, but you like the team approach and the creativity involved with meeting each person's safety and health needs, while discovering and supporting each one's unique personality.

You heard at the Monday morning team meeting that a new resident named Samuel Duncan was going to be admitted today. He and his wife have been living in the independent housing area of the retirement community, and Mr. Duncan has attended the day program for the past 3 years. You want to meet with Mr. Duncan and his wife today to learn about his personal care routines so you can match them as closely as possible to help preserve his independence. This is especially important during the critical adjustment phase after admission. You log into the electronic documentation program used by the Living Center to learn more about Samuel Duncan.

In the demographic area of the record you see that Mr. Duncan is 65 years old, is African American, and his religious affiliation is listed as Methodist. The couple has long-term-care insurance that pays for any long-term-care medical expenses. In the medical report, you learn that Mr. Duncan was diagnosed with Alzheimer's disease when he was only 52 years old. In addition to Alzheimer's disease, Samuel Duncan has sickle cell anemia and rheumatoid arthritis that has recently impacted his fine motor coordination. He is on Aricept for his dementia, and hydroxyurea for sickle cell anemia. He also takes naproxen sodium for his arthritis pain.

The latest progress notes from the day program give you some insight into why Mr. Duncan is being admitted to the dementia unit. Due to his confusion he has become increasingly paranoid, suspecting that others are taking his items or hiding them on him. He has had several incidents over the past 2 months of hitting the other residents and staff at the day program, pulling at their clothing, and becoming very upset and anxious. He is quite strong, and has also begun trying to wheel himself outside. His wife is quite distraught at moving Mr. Duncan into the skilled facility, but she reports that he gets up frequently at night, tries to go outside, and becomes physically aggressive sometimes when she tries to help him with personal care.

You look for other clues in the information provided, getting a sense of what his "normal" routine is, and what he responds and reacts to. You note that he is an early riser, is more cooperative in the morning, and is most anxious and difficult to manage in the evenings and at night. In the past he always enjoyed being outside and talking with his neighbors. At the day program, his favorite activities were helping take care of the plants and watching old movies. When he becomes anxious, the triggers seem to be when someone is trying to "rush" him, or when there is a lot of noise and confusion. Calming activities include going for a ride in his wheelchair especially outside, and sitting in a rocking chair near a window.

You go down to the nurses' station and talk to the nursing care aide assigned to Mr. Duncan to ask how he is doing. She smiles and says he and his wife are nice people, and Mrs. Duncan seems to be really good with him. She tells you no one is with them right now, and it would probably be a good time to see him. You pick up a hunting and a gardening magazine on your way down the hall, and knock on Mr. Duncan's door. When his wife says, "Come in," you enter and introduce yourself. The room, like all of them on the dementia unit, is private. This reduces the noise and confusion, and minimizes conflict between residents. You are glad to see that Mrs. Duncan has already brought some personal furnishings to the room for Mr. Duncan. He is a small black man, sitting in a recliner that looks too big for him. He is dressed neatly in a fresh, white button-down shirt and khaki pants. He is gazing out the window with a furrowed brow. You introduce yourself, and tell Mr. Duncan you brought him some magazines. He looks at you but doesn't smile. When you put the magazines in front of him, he opens the top one and begins to flip the pages. Mrs. Duncan turns away from her husband and tells you quietly that she hopes she is not making a mistake. "I just don't know what is going to happen when he realizes he is not going home with me tonight." She starts to cry and says, "This is the first time we will be apart overnight in many years."

Questions as You Begin

Consider these questions as you begin developing this case:

- You realize that this is a big change for both of the Duncans, and you feel bad that Mrs. Duncan is so upset. You would like to help her as well. Your referral for treatment though is for Mr. Duncan. What is your obligation to his wife in this situation?
- You understand her concern about what will happen when he understands that he is going to stay at the nursing facility and not return home. Who is the right person to tell him this?

Congenital Neurologic Conditions

The next two cases present congenital neurologic conditions; a child in a school setting and an adult living at a group residence. In both cases, the therapist is working with the individual in his or her natural environment, and helping the client engage in social and productive occupations with peers. Congenital neurologic conditions are unique in that they are present from birth, and individuals may need treatment and special support at key phases of development throughout their lives.

The therapist is in the role of providing *habilitation* or establishing skills as opposed to *re*habilitation where we seek to restore or remediate limitations in functioning. When introducing new performance skills, whether they are motor, process, or social interaction skills, the aim is to allow your client to participate in age-appropriate and meaningful occupations and activities. It is equally important to incorporate the learning process into the natural setting as much as possible to improve generalization of the skill.[7]

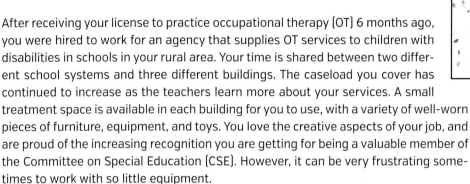

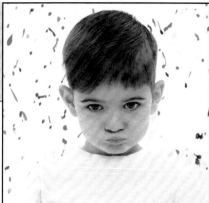

CASE 4.10

CLIENT:	Theodore Lindstrom, 6-year-old Caucasian male
CONDITION:	Spina bifida
SETTING:	School-based services

After receiving your license to practice occupational therapy (OT) 6 months ago, you were hired to work for an agency that supplies OT services to children with disabilities in schools in your rural area. Your time is shared between two different school systems and three different buildings. The caseload you cover has continued to increase as the teachers learn more about your services. A small treatment space is available in each building for you to use, with a variety of well-worn pieces of furniture, equipment, and toys. You love the creative aspects of your job, and are proud of the increasing recognition you are getting for being a valuable member of the Committee on Special Education (CSE). However, it can be very frustrating sometimes to work with so little equipment.

This morning you received a note that a new student just transferred to one of your schools and needs to be evaluated for services. A CSE meeting has been set for 1 month from today in order to allow time for evaluations to be completed. Most of the school systems in your area use an electronic database and recordkeeping system that makes information transfer between schools relatively seamless. You are hopeful that the information from the prior school has been transferred and that a new case file for your district is available for viewing. On your lunch break you finally have time to get online. You are pleased when you find background medical as well as educational and personal information.

Theodore (known as "Teddy") is 6 years and 4 months of age, and was born with a myelomeningocele, or Spina Bifida. As with many children born with this condition, Teddy also had hydrocephalus. This symptom was discovered shortly after birth and a shunt was placed immediately. His shunt was replaced twice since birth due to malfunctions. Teddy's deficits from the congenital malformation include paralysis and lack of sensation in his lower trunk, legs and feet, mild scoliosis, and decreased fine motor skills. He is significantly below the median height and weight for his age. Teddy also suffers from asthma, which is controlled with medications.

Teddy is the youngest of three children. He was placed in foster care when 3 months old by his mother, after his father abandoned the family. Teddy's mother took the two older children and moved out of the area, expressing no interest in having further contact with Teddy. Child Protective Services have been unable to clear him for adoption as a special-needs child. He has been moved several times to different foster homes. You can't tell from the record why he was moved this time.

Teddy attends a Spina Bifida clinic quarterly, and reports from the clinic are also included in the confidential file from the most recent visit. You note that Teddy's scoliosis appears to be stable, with no increase in the spinal curvature over the past two quarters. He has a reciprocating gait orthosis (RGO) and the clinic recommends that this be used at least twice daily for standing activities. His skin integrity is good with no history of pressure areas.

Previous school assessments show that Teddy has difficulty with independent transfers and has delays in dressing and toileting skills. He is able to move around the classroom using a manual wheelchair, but needs to be pushed for longer distances. He is able to feed himself after setup, and his reading and handwriting skills are slightly below age level. He was in the first grade at his previous school, and you note that your school has placed him with a very experienced first-grade teacher. The records also indicate that he needs some assistance while at school with wheelchair mobility between rooms as well as toileting, managing clothes, and meal setup. He has been noted by the previous school psychologist to have anger management issues and low self-esteem. He is manipulative with adults and often does not get along well with peers. You find a separate entry dated 2 days ago from your school nurse that Teddy has a prescription for Pulmacort and a rescue inhaler for asthma and Bactrim for a urinary tract infection (UTI).

Teddy's most recent Individualized Education Plan (IEP) from his previous school outlines a plan for wheelchair accessibility, levels of assistance, and adaptations necessary to support his participation and performance. This educational plan indicates that Teddy had previously received physical therapy to work on transfers and mobility, and occupational therapy to work on handwriting, and social skills. There were also psychology services in his IEP with goals to address self-esteem issues and coping skills. You wonder which discipline incorporated use of the RGO into treatment, and why the OT didn't have any occupational performance goals related to independence in self-care skills.

You make arrangements to see Teddy to begin your initial assessment 2 days later during his class' gym time. A teacher's aide brings Teddy to your room. You observe that he is wearing faded jeans, and a white tee shirt. He is seated in a special wheelchair and looks younger than 6 years. When the aide leaves and tells Teddy that she will be back in a half hour, the child does not respond. You introduce yourself and he looks at you but does not say anything. You ask him to tell you about the occupational therapist at his last school and what kinds of activities he liked. Teddy tells you that the OT was "dumb," and wanted him to play "baby games." When you ask him to tell you about his favorite thing to do in school, he quickly says painting, but then changes his mind and says he prefers to go to the library where the "mean kids won't bug me." Next, you ask him about what he likes to do when he's not at school, and he tells you he likes to watch TV and read story books.

Questions as You Begin

Consider these questions as you begin developing this case:

- If Teddy has a history of being manipulative with adults, and anger management issues, what is the best approach to take with him on this first day?
- Being moved, not just to a new school but to a whole new family, must be really hard for a 6-year-old. It seems like letting him express how he feels about all this might be beneficial. How could you incorporate that into an activity that would also address one of his identified needs such as fine motor skills?

CASE 4.11	CLIENT:	Sarah Morgan, 32-year-old Caucasian female
	CONDITION:	Down syndrome
	SETTING:	Independent contractor serving community residences for cognitively impaired clients

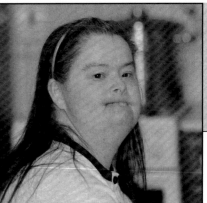

You provide occupational therapy services as an independent contractor to an agency that serves the adult developmentally disabled population. This non-profit agency operates both residential and day habilitation services in a variety of locations throughout a three-county area. Most of your referrals come from the staff in the residential homes. The homes are located in neighborhoods throughout the region, with small groups of 8 to 15 residents living in each. The residents are admitted to one of the homes based on the amount of assistance and medical needs they have, with the number of support staff matched to the level of care. Although residents will occasionally be moved between houses if their conditions decline, staff and residents frequently form social bonds, and there is usually a strong preference to manage residents with creative interventions and problem solving instead of moving them.

You are called on to assess and make recommendations for a variety of issues, including environmental adaptations, adaptive equipment and mobility needs, developing personal care routines, and problem-solving challenges with social, leisure, and productivity issues. You love the fact that every challenge is unique and different. Many times your ability to design client-centered solutions can make a world of difference for both staff and residents.

Today you have been asked to visit a small home on Adams Street where 12 residents live. The criteria to live in this home is that residents have to be able to ambulate independently or use a mobility device unassisted, must need no more than minimal assistance for dressing and toileting and moderate assistance for bathing, and attend a workshop or day habilitation setting during the week. You arrive at the home shortly before the residents return from their day programs. There are only a few staff and they are not able to sit with you right then. They explain to you that they are concerned about one of the newer residents named Sarah Morgan. While you wait for one of them to get freed up to talk, you ask for this resident's chart to get some background information. Sarah is a 32-year-old Caucasian female. She was born with Down syndrome and has a moderate to severe intellectual impairment with an intelligence quotient (IQ) measured at 35. Other symptoms related to her diagnosis are impaired vision corrected with glasses, a large and protruding tongue, congenital heart disease resulting in cardiomyopathy, and poor immune function. Sarah is taking Atenolol and Lasix to manage her heart condition. She has had several severe episodes of pneumonia.

In the family history portion of the chart you see that Sarah has three much older siblings, and her parents are both deceased. She lived at home with her parents until she was 12 years, and then with an older sister until she was 18 years. Sarah was in a 6-1-1 classroom at school until the age of 18. Her family then transferred Sarah to one of the residences run by your agency. Sarah's family has remained involved, calling once a week and taking her out on "field trips" to family holidays and activities.

She was transferred to the Adams Street home from another residence with the same agency that was several miles away. Sarah's previous home had to be closed because the property could no longer meet the new building code requirements. Staff members were not sure Sarah was suited for the Adams Street home at first because she was on the edge of needing more care than they could offer. However, it was documented that she seemed to take to the staff easily, and Sarah's family had really pushed for the placement saying it was close to her sister's home, and she would be able to continue at the same-day habilitation program. The staff had been able to arrange for Sarah to visit the new home a few times before the move, and one of the other residents from her previous home was also moved to the Adams Street home along with Sarah.

Two staff members come to sit with you to talk about why they have asked for your assistance with Sarah. They tell you that Sarah has a cheerful disposition most of the time, and usually gets along well with other residents. For the most part she has settled into the home's routines. She has dysarthria but she is able to communicate simple needs. Like many of the residents she has difficulty understanding or expressing abstract ideas. Sarah likes routines and everything in its place. Sometimes conflict arises when other residents do not follow the routines and Sarah becomes upset. When this happens she will usually make loud angry noises and cry until it is corrected. Sometimes she will become quite stubborn by sitting down on the floor when something is not going the way she thinks it should.

The latest challenge that had caused the staff to ask you for assistance is concern over Sarah's behavior related to the kitchen. Sarah has seen several of the residents who are at a higher occupational performance level going into the kitchen and either making their lunches or doing small tasks to help prepare the evening meal. Sarah does not have "kitchen privileges" since there are not enough staff to work one-on-one with her in the kitchen. The staff have tried to distract her at these times with other activities she enjoys like puzzles and magazines, but this has not been effective. They have also tried to have her work with another resident to set napkins around the table, thinking that she would be involved in the meal process, but she has not been willing to do this either. When she is asked to leave the kitchen, she becomes angry and lately has started to grab at the food and utensils. Two days ago she received a minor cut when she grabbed a butter knife away from another resident in the kitchen. The staff are looking for assistance from you, and tell you they are at their wit's end. Sarah is at the lower end of the criteria to live at the home, and they are wondering if perhaps she would be better suited at another home where there are more staff, and more of the residents function at a lower level similar to Sarah's. They know it is hard on the residents when they move, and they would prefer to work things out here at the Adams Street home so that she can be safe and happy here. You ask what her favorite activities are and they tell you she loves music, looking at pictures of her with her family, going through magazines, and doing puzzles with animals.

Just then the bus arrives with the residents. The staff are quickly caught up in the activity as everyone comes in at once. Sarah is pointed out to you and you approach her to introduce yourself. She is a short, stocky woman who moves with purpose toward a closet. Although you say "Hello!" as she passes by you, she does not pause or look up, but continues to her destination. You watch as she puts her shoes and coat in the closet, making sure all the shoes are straight. After she closes the door she takes a bag and heads toward the kitchen. One of the staff asks her where she is going and she stops and looks at the staff warily. She looks at the bag in her hand, and then heads for the kitchen again. One staff member goes with her, telling her, "Let's get a snack and take it out to the table." This seems to pacify Sarah and she happily piles some crackers and cheese that are handed to her onto a plate. She seems reluctant to leave the room, and watches two other residents making their lunches for the next day. One of them comes near her and asks her to move so he can get a spoon. She looks back angrily and says, "No!" and refuses to move. Finally, the staff member convinces her that she has to come out to the dining room to eat her snack.

You sit with the staff in an adjacent room for a few more minutes to brainstorm about Sarah. One of them tells you that what you had just witnessed was a good example of the problem, because it could have continued to escalate in the kitchen. You ask them what they think she wants to do in the kitchen–is she actually trying to get food to eat? Both of them agree that she does not actually seem to be hungry or trying to eat food, but it seems to be more about a desire to engage in the preparation of food. You wonder if somehow making her own lunch seems like a status symbol to Sarah, or perhaps just a desire to do what she sees others doing.

You decide to talk to some staff who used to work at Sarah's previous home to find out what association, if any, Sarah might have had with preparing food. By the next day you are able to reach an aide who knows Sarah from her old home . He tells you that helping staff in the kitchen was a privilege that one resident had each dinner time. Tasks consisted of simple tasks such as carrying things to the table, putting items on a tray, or mixing something with supervision and assistance as needed. There were typically two staff in the kitchen with one resident. The aide tells you that Sarah seemed to look forward to her turn to help, and they had not had problems with Sarah trying to take things from others or going into the kitchen when it was not her turn. There had only been 10 residents at that home, and most had been similar to Sarah in cognitive ability.

Questions as You Begin

Consider these questions as you begin developing this case:

- You can appreciate the staff's concern for Sarah and the other residents' safety, but you wonder why they couldn't spend some one-on-one time in the kitchen with Sarah every day. It seems like they should have enough staff to do this, but they have pretty much said, "This house is not set up for that." If it is in the client's best interest, and they have the staff to do it, how can you get the policy and/or staff's attitude changed?

REFERENCES

1. Brasure M, Lamberty GJ, Sayer NA, et al. Multidisciplinary Postacute Rehabilitation for Moderate to Severe Traumatic Brain Injury in Adults. Comparative Effectiveness Review No. 72. (Prepared by the Minnesota Evidence-based Practice Center under Contract No. HHSA-290-2007-10064-I.) AHRQ Publication No. 12-EHC101-EF. Rockville, MD: Agency for Healthcare Research and Quality; June 2012. www.effectivehealth-care.ahrq.gov/reports/final.cfm.

2. Ashley M. A Review of Efforts to Prevent and Treat Traumatic Brain Injury. Testimony of Mark J. Ashley, Sc.D., CCC-SLP, CCM Chairman Emeritus, Brain Injury Association of America. Lecture conducted for Subcommittee on Health, Committee on Energy and Commerce; March 19, 2012; Washington, DC.

3. Teasdale G, Jennett B. Assessment of coma and impaired consciousness: a practical scale. *Lancet.* 1974;304(7872):81–84.

4. Keith RA, Granger CV, Hamilton BB, et al. The functional independence measure: a new tool for rehabilitation. *Adv Clin Rehabil.* 1987;1:6–18.

5. Brown A, Kern R. Disease adaptation may have decreased quality-of-life responsiveness in patients with chronic progressive neurological disorders. *J Clin Epidemiol.* 2004;57:1033–1039.

6. Engstrom B, Norberg A, Nordeson A. Self-reported quality of life for patients with progressive neurological diseases. *Qual Life Res.* 1998;7:257–266.

7. Stone-MacDonald A. Learning daily life and vocational skills in natural settings: a Tanzanian model. *J Int Assoc Spec Educ.* 2012;13:28–40.

Cardiopulmonary Cases

Although most therapists who work with clients with cardiopulmonary conditions do so in an acute care setting, there is much value that an occupational therapist (OT) could add in the outpatient cardiac rehabilitation and home settings as well. Concepts of energy conservation, metabolic equivalent of tasks or MET levels, and monitoring vitals during occupational performance are all introduced in the hospital, immediately following a cardiopulmonary health crisis. But much of this early recovery time with conditions such as myocardial infarctions is overwhelmed by uncertainty, activity restriction, anxiety, and depression.[1] How much more effective might it be if we were able to accompany our clients through their transition back into the community?

As our profession continues to move away from a medical model and toward a broader and more holistic vision, the overarching statement describing our domain seems to speak so perfectly to the needs of so many of our clients with cardiopulmonary conditions:

"Achieving health, well-being, and participation in life through engagement in occupation."

AOTA, 2014[2]

CASE

5.1

CLIENT: Elena Gomez, 52-year-old Caucasian female

CONDITION: Myocardial infarction with CABG

SETTING: Hospital inpatient cardiac unit

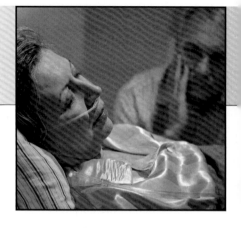

You have just received an order from the inpatient cardiac unit of the hospital to evaluate and treat Elena Gomez. Her primary diagnosis listed on the referral is acute myocardial infarction (MI). You also note on the referral that she is 52 years old, and was admitted to the intensive care unit (ICU) 3 days ago. You review the chart and see on the basic intake form that she weighs 170 pounds and is 5 ft 2 in tall, is originally from Puerto Rico, and speaks Spanish as her first language, but is fluent in English as well. Her health insurance is Excellus, through her employer. Her history and physical report dictated by the admitting physician indicate that she has a history of high blood pressure, but no previous history of MI. The note from the emergency department (ED) on admission states that she awoke from a sound sleep with crushing chest pain four nights ago and was transported to the hospital after her husband called for an ambulance.

After running a variety of tests in the ED, Mrs. Gomez was sent to the catheterization lab and a heart catheterization was performed. The report indicated a 90% blockage of the left anterior descending coronary artery, and Mrs. Gomez was taken to the operating room for emergency cardiac surgery. The operating room report indicates that she received a coronary artery bypass graft (CABG) on two of her heart vessels without complications. She has spent the past 3 days in the intensive care unit following surgery. The patient has been placed on sternal precautions, and the physician has set her cardiac target not to exceed 60% of maximum heart rate during activities.

You also notice that her medical history indicates that she has received long-term treatment with medication for anxiety. Physician progress notes from the first 3 days of her hospital stay state that she has progressed well since surgery with no complications other than her anxiety, which has been higher than normal, and is felt to be aggravating her current cardiac status. Today's medical progress note states that she is now medically stable and will be transferred out to the inpatient cardiac unit. Physical therapy and occupational therapy were both ordered to begin today with Phase I of the hospital's cardiac rehabilitation program.

On her list of medications you note that she is on Plavix and Simvastatin for her cardiac problems, and an increased dose of Ativan for her anxiety, with Clonazepam ordered as needed (PRN) for increases in anxiety. Nursing notes indicate that she is responding well with improved cardiac rhythms and a slight reduction in anxiety as evidenced by reduced restlessness and fewer requests for help. The incision from surgery is healing well, and the patient continues on sternal precautions. The social work note states that she lives with her 65-year-old husband, and has one teenaged child still at home, and two other adult children who live nearby and are attentive. The discharge plan is for her to return home with community services and referral to the hospital's level II cardiac rehabilitation program. You note that physical therapy has completed their assessment, and are recommending a two-person assist for transfer, and a standard walker to be used in the client's room.

You visit Mrs. Gomez briefly in her room to introduce yourself. She is sitting in a bedside chair and attempting to eat her lunch, but she tells you she feels weak and does not want to eat. There are several family members in the room speaking rapidly in Spanish and taking turns trying to coax her to eat. Her room is filled with cards and several bouquets of flowers. Mrs. Gomez is tearful and appears anxious during your short visit. She tells you that she has four grandchildren and she enjoys knitting and cooking. She works as a clerk for a local law office part time, but she tells you she will probably have to give that up now. Her husband worked for the railroad and has a good pension and private health insurance, but now he suffers from arthritis in his back and is not able to do much around the house. The couple lives in a large two-story home where they have raised their children on the outskirts of a small town in this rural community. She tells you that her husband just told her he wants to put their house up for sale and move into something smaller because the housework is too much for her. She tells you, "I feel like my life is ending, even though I survived the heart attack."

Questions as You Begin

Consider these questions as you begin developing this case:

- Mrs. Gomez is being faced with some big decisions about her job and home. You wonder if this isn't adding to the anxiety she is feeling. How can you get her husband and family to delay these discussions until Mrs. Gomez is farther along in her recovery?
- How can you help her manage her anxiety as you begin working with her on cardiac rehabilitation?
- You are also worried about her fresh cardiac status and pushing her too hard. How do you know how hard to push her?

CASE

5.2

CLIENT: Brandon Greer, 48-year-old Caucasian male

CONDITION: AIDS-related pneumonia

SETTING: Hospital inpatient cardiopulmonary unit; hospice residence

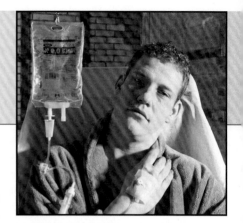

Initial Setting

You work in a regional healthcare center with many specialty clinics. About 3 months ago you transferred from the outpatient rehabilitation clinic to the inpatient clinic when there was an opening. You really enjoy the camaraderie of the therapists you work with in your new job. One of the things you like most is how the interprofessional team works together with different disciplines. Each OT is assigned to an interprofessional team made up of the nurses on a particular unit, the hospitalist assigned to that unit, and a physical and occupational therapist, social worker, dietitian, and sometimes others. For example, your team provides service primarily to clients on the cardiopulmonary unit so there is also a respiratory therapist (RT) on your team.

The entire interprofessional team meets briefly in the morning and receives report from the charge nurse and hospitalist to review the status of each patient on the unit, discuss progress and discharge plans, and ask questions about any new admissions. This morning you learn that there is a new admission to the unit. He is a 48-year-old male named Brandon Greer admitted with a severe case of pneumocystis pneumonia (PCP) secondary to HIV infection. He is on social security disability with Medicare Parts A and B insurance coverage. The hospitalist is very concerned about this patient's critical status, and says his hope is that the patient's condition will improve so that he can be discharged back home with his partner and in-home services. However, the doctor is worried because Mr. Greer is refusing a variety of the more aggressive treatments he has suggested. The social worker confirms that Mr. Greer has been living with HIV for many years, and has grown discouraged with the side effects of treatments and his current quality of life. He had to retire from his job as a magazine editor about 6 months ago because of his health. The nurse shares that Mr. Greer's partner has been instrumental in convincing him to at least continue taking Tenofovir, an antiretroviral medication that he has been prescribed as well as Bactrim to combat the pneumonia.

The history of the present illness is that his CD4 cell count had dropped to around 50 before he went to his doctor and got started on the Bactrim. The physician tells the care team that he suspects the patient had not been taking his antiretroviral medications as regularly as prescribed, but regardless, his immunosuppressed state made him vulnerable to this particular type of pneumonia. His current symptoms include shortness of breath (SOB), intermittent fever, dry cough, rapid breathing, chest pain, and fatigue. He is currently on continuous oxygen to address his hypoxia and intravenous antibiotics for the pneumonia. The nurse mentions that although Mr. Greer has requested to be on "Do Not Resuscitate" status, his partner has expressed concern that the patient is depressed, and might feel differently if the depression were treated. The physician says he will explore this with the patient.

The rehabilitation members of the team are requested to try to prevent further deconditioning through light activity, and to explore quality of life issues to see if there are ways to balance the impact of treatment options with life satisfaction. You talk with the physical therapist (PT) on the team after the meeting and agree that you will meet with Mr. Greer during lunch, and then the PT will visit later in the day. The social worker stops you and the dietitian as you are leaving the meeting to tell you that she has discovered that Mr. Greer has a sweet tooth, loves good food and fine wine, and loves to travel. She says she doesn't know if this information will help you, but she thought she would pass it on. You ask the dietitian about dietary restrictions for Mr. Greer and she tells you, "He has lost so much weight at this point, anything he wants to eat he can have! And push fluids if you have the chance."

When you go in to see Mr. Greer you find him in bed. He looks pale, tired, and discouraged. Another man sits nearby, talking quietly with him. You introduce yourself and the patient acknowledges you, but doesn't speak. You explain what you do, and wait for a response. He tells you, "I'm not sure if I have enough energy to do anything. But I know I'm tired of being a burden on Joseph here." Just then the lunch tray is delivered. Joseph encourages him to try to eat, and offers to feed him. The patient just shakes his head and looks away. Joseph tells you, "Maybe I'll take a walk, and let you two get acquainted."

Questions as You Begin

Consider these questions as you begin developing this case:

- This is the first time you have treated an HIV-positive patient since you took this job. What are your personal feelings about working with Mr. Greer?
- Do you have any personal biases that may affect your work with him?
- How can you address personal biases?
- Mr. Greer's partner plays an important role in his health care. How can you include him either directly or indirectly?
- Should you talk with the client about depression, or leave that to the physician?

Transfer to Hospice Residence

You work as an independent contractor, filling in per diem for several outpatient facilities, providing service twice a week at a small private nursing home, and consulting with a local hospice residence. You love the flexibility of your practice, and being your own boss. Your work at the hospice involves meeting with residents and a team of staff that specializes in end-of-life care to adjust personal care routines and various aspects of life to help residents not only be comfortable, but to achieve a balance between care and quality of life. Although your job here can be emotionally difficult, it is deeply satisfying to know that you often help people find comfort and even satisfaction and joy during the end stage of their lives. Admission to the home is limited to persons who have been certified by their physician as being terminally ill, with a prognosis of 6 months or less if the disease runs its natural course. In addition, the individual must have made the decision to forego further curative treatment. The focus of care is on enriching residents' lives and helping them achieve physical comfort, and emotional, social, and spiritual well-being. Medicare Part A and some private insurances will help pay toward the cost of services provided at the residence.

You received a call yesterday that there was a new resident at the hospice. You don't have remote access to the medical records of the facility, so you have to wait until you get to the house this afternoon to find out more. As you enter the long driveway you admire the house, a one-storey residence located in a quiet neighborhood on a large, wooded lot. It has been converted so that up to six people can live in the facility at a time. Each private room has an adjoining, private bath and a small attached room that doubles as both a sitting area to visit privately with others, or a guest bedroom if loved ones wish to stay. A large open kitchen and great room with a fireplace are in the middle, opening onto a back deck. Additional rooms include a large family-style dining room, a small office, and a locked medication room. Staff at the facility all have special training in hospice care and include hospice nurses who specialize in pain and symptom management for the terminally ill, personal care aides, a social worker, a part-time dietitian, several cooks and cleaning staff, and a Medical Director.

You use your pass key to enter and pass through the entry way to the office where you find the nursing director, known by everyone as Louie. He greets you with a smile and pulls a chair out so you can join him at the desk. Between Louie's briefing and the chart, you learn that Brandon Greer was admitted yesterday, with end-stage AIDS. He has been treated for HIV for almost 20 years, and has made the decision to stop further aggressive treatment after a recent hospitalization for AIDS-related pneumonia. His longtime partner, Joseph Deal, is struggling to come to terms with this decision. The hospital social worker and Mr. Greer's primary physician spent a lot of time with both of them, and Louie tells you that it was Mr. Greer's choice to come to the house rather than seeking hospice care at home. Louie says, "He told Joseph he wanted to spend his remaining days enjoying time with him, not having Joe care for him." You noted in the chart that end-of-life paperwork had been completed, giving Joe power-of-attorney and appointing him as healthcare agent.

You see that an OT worked with Mr. Greer in the hospital. The discharge note from the therapist states that he worked on using adaptive equipment for dressing, bathing, and grooming, and incorporating energy conservation techniques into his personal care routines. Mr. Greer is on continuous oxygen, and needs one assist to ambulate short distances with a wheeled walker. Since admission to the hospice house, Louie tells you that his major symptoms are shortness of breath, anxiety, and some nausea. He has not been in a lot of pain so far, and they have not had to use the Morphine ordered "as needed" by the medical director. Mr. Greer had chosen to discontinue taking the antiretroviral medication. He is now taking Ativan for anxiety and Zofran for the nausea. "The trick," Louie notes, "is going to be to keep him comfortable but alert so he can enjoy things." You note his past interests listed on the hospital OT summary: gourmet food and travel.

You use the in-house intercom system to buzz Mr. Greer's room. You hear him cough and then ask who it is. After giving your name and asking if you can see him, you are invited to come back to his room. The door is opened by a large man with a worried look on his face. He introduces himself as Joseph, Brandon's partner. After exchanging greetings you see the resident reclining in a comfortable chair, a glass of wine on a table next to him. "Please, come in and join us" you are told.

Questions as You Begin

Consider these questions as you begin developing this case:

- The therapist in this case is challenged yet inspired by working with patients on hospice care. How do you feel about working with this patient population?
- You may face the prospect of a client of yours dying, in many different practice settings. What can you do to prepare yourself to deal with this aspect of care effectively?

CLIENT: Boris Schneider, 68-year-old Caucasian male

CONDITION: Chronic obstructive pulmonary disease

SETTING: Homecare agency

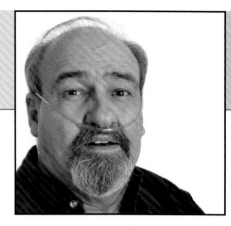

You work for a homecare agency in a rural area. You see clients with a variety of conditions, both postacute and chronic. Usually when you go to see a new referral for the first time, the nurse case manager has already made at least one visit. Sometimes a PT has also completed an initial evaluation, and information from your colleagues is available on a private computer network for your review before your visit. Today you see that you have received a new order to see Boris Schneider, a 68-year-old man referred by Dr. Atwell, his primary care physician. Mr. Schneider has just been discharged from the local hospital for an exacerbation of chronic obstructive pulmonary disease (COPD). You log onto another area of the network to get some additional information. Under demographic data, you find that he lives with his wife in a rural area, home to a large German population. His occupation is listed as "retired cabinetmaker." His religious affiliation is listed as Jewish. He is covered by Medicare insurance, Part A and Part B.

The accompanying discharge information from the hospital reveals that he was discharged after a 10-day hospital stay for a respiratory infection and exacerbation of his COPD, with an order to continue on long-term oxygen therapy (LTOT). His recovery had several setbacks, and multiple medications were tried before his respiratory status began to improve. By time of discharge home, the hospital physical therapy note states that Mr. Schneider was walking 100 ft three times per day with supervision, using continuous oxygen at 2 litres per minute. The occupational therapy discharge note indicates he was able to feed himself after setup and was bathing and dressing his upper body with supervision. He needed minimal assistance using adaptive equipment to bathe and dress his lower body. All activities of daily living (ADLs) were performed with oxygen therapy in use. Information stated that the client has indicated that his goal is to return to driving and taking care of things around the house as soon as possible. His recreational interests include home maintenance and playing poker with his friends. He has asked for a portable oxygen tank for home use, in addition to an oxygen concentrator.

The social work note from the hospital indicates that he has a wife, Gertrude, at home and a son who lives nearby. Mr. Schneider and his wife both immigrated with their parents to the area as children. German is their primary language, although both speak English well, but with a heavy accent. Mr. Schneider has smoked one pack of cigarettes a day for many years. He has always handled all of the family finances and has done most of the driving. The nursing discharge summary indicates that the patient's wife is nervous about taking him home because he is "bull headed" and doesn't listen. She also fears he will not stay on his diet, refrain from smoking, or follow his doctor's orders restricting his physical activity including driving. Dr. Atwell recommended that Mr. Schneider receive home therapy for reconditioning, and to learn more energy conservation methods. His discharge medications are Levaquin for the respiratory infection and Advair, a bronchodilator.

The homecare case was initiated by a nurse case manager. Referrals have been made for both OT and PT to go into the home. The initial homecare nursing note indicates that Mr. Schneider's respiratory status was essentially stable since discharge from the hospital. He expressed anger about his condition and his restrictions on smoking and diet, but was generally cooperative with the nurse. The nurse helped the family set up the client's medications in a pill organizer, and reviewed each medicine with him and his wife as well as the need for the doctor's recommended restrictions. The physical therapy note states that the client appeared to have been quite sedentary since returning home, and became short of breath after only 25 ft even with the use of oxygen at 2 litres. A home exercise program was given to Mr. Schneider by the PT to increase strength and endurance.

You find Mr. Schneider and his wife in the kitchen when you arrive, and he is watching her prepare a meal. He is wearing a robe over pajamas even though it is 1:00 PM, he is receiving oxygen from a concentrator nearby, and he does not look happy. Mrs. Schneider encourages you to join them at the kitchen table and offers you strong black coffee. Mr. Schneider is quick to get right to business saying, "I don't know what you can do that the other young PT fella can't. I'm not happy about things and that's all there is to it!" Mrs. Schneider sighs and rolls her eyes, scolding him for being rude to the nice therapist. "I would think you would show a little appreciation to all the people that are working hard to keep you at home!"

You see that Mr. Schneider had been working on a crossword puzzle. You decide to try a direct approach. "Okay, Mr. Schneider, you say you are not happy about things? Then let's talk. What do you want to be able to do? Let's tackle it together." Mrs. Schneider stops what she is doing to see how he will respond. Mr. Schneider quietly answers, "I want to fix that broken wall light in the hallway. And I want to take a shower by myself!"

Questions as You Begin

Consider these questions as you begin developing this case:

- It sounds like Mr. Schneider can get very difficult when he is frustrated or angry. You think about your own personality, and how you usually respond when faced with someone like this. Would that response be the best approach with Mr. Schneider to meet his needs?
- How can you improve your ability to respond differently?
- How will he accept having a female work with him on showering?
- What can you do to make this more comfortable for him?

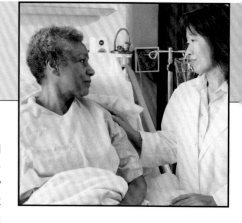

CASE

5.4

CLIENT: Loretta Thompson, 74-year-old African
                American female

CONDITION: Congestive heart failure

SETTING: Hospital inpatient cardiopulmonary unit

University hospital sits on a hill overlooking a small college town in a rural area. You work in the rehabilitation department and are assigned primarily to the inpatient units. Occasionally, if the inpatient census is low, you help out in the attached nursing home or the outpatient clinic. You always check your case assignment first thing in the morning. Today you see that you have six medical and postsurgical inpatients who will need revisits, and one new referral for the cardiopulmonary unit. Your assignment sheet for the day provides minimal information about new cases. The only information on the new client is her name, Loretta Thompson, 74 years old, with an admission diagnosis of congestive heart failure.

You know that you will find a lot more information on Ms. Thompson in the electronic medical record on the hospital's proprietary electronic database. There is only a half hour before you need to start your inpatient treatments, so you use the time to log on and get to know more about Loretta Thompson. On the demographic information page, you find that she is from Haiti and speaks English and Creole. Under marital status it says divorced. There is no mention of a religious affiliation. Under employment status it says "shop owner." Her insurance coverage is listed as Medicare Parts A and B with an additional supplemental insurance.

The social work admission note gives you a lot more information about your new patient's personal context. It states that Ms. Thompson emigrated from Haiti when she was 40 to escape a "bad marriage." Ten years later she became an American citizen. She is a woman of medium build who speaks with a strong accent. She is 74 years old, although she appears much younger. She owns a small store in town selling "cultural artifacts," and works long hours. She has a handyman who comes in a few times a week to help her, but she still does a lot of the work herself. She eats sporadically, cooking on a hotpot in the back room. She states she has seven children, but some of them are adopted from other family members. Several of these children still reside in Haiti apparently, and others live in various parts of the United States. She occasionally has grandchildren who will stay with her for a time, but she states she has no relatives living in the area at this time.

In the medical history and physical report, you note that she was admitted to the cardiac unit after being brought to the ED by ambulance when someone found her barely conscious on the floor in her store. On admission to the ED, she was confused but moving all four extremities. Pitting edema was noted in both lower extremities. An electrocardiogram (ECG) in the ED showed bradycardia and her blood pressure was low. Oxygen therapy and transcutaneous pacing were provided, and Lasix was started to reduce the buildup of fluid.

The initial medical note after admission to the hospital indicated that Ms. Thompson's cognitive status was improving and she supplied the information that she does not smoke or drink, but has a history of very high cholesterol and high blood pressure. She has had edema in both lower extremities for quite some time, and complains of heaviness in her chest starting 2 days ago. She has no primary physician and goes to a "friend" when she needs health care, preferring homeopathic health interventions.

A follow-up social work note on the day after admission indicates that Mrs. Thompson has a large group of friends in the community with many visitors coming to the hospital already. Several visitors have identified themselves as relatives of Ms. Thompson, but their relationship to the patient is unclear. The nursing staff has complained that the visitors are loud, and are bringing food in to Ms. Thompson, which makes it difficult to measure input and output of fluids and nutrition. The patient has shared that she loves to play cards with her friends and cook traditional foods. She has certain TV shows that she never misses. Her plans are to return to her tiny one-bedroom apartment and continue to run her store. She reluctantly told the social worker that she will arrange for more assistance at the store, but she has not been willing thus far to accept the idea of referrals for any services at home such as meals on wheels or a visiting nurse program.

Since her admission to the cardiac unit, Atenolol and Digoxin have been prescribed to further stabilize her cardiac status. She has responded well to treatment and is now on day 2 of admission. The cardiologist has recommended that she begin rehabilitation, with the target range between 50% and 85% of her maximum heart rate (MHR). The discharge plan is to her home, but she lives alone and the physician is concerned about her ability to manage independently, given the chronic nature of her condition and the lifestyle changes that will be necessary to maintain her health. Occupational therapy has been asked to evaluate her functional status and provide input to the interprofessional team regarding requirements for a safe discharge.

After lunch you head up to the cardiac unit to begin the evaluation with Ms. Thompson. The door is open and you find three visitors in the room speaking rapidly in a heavily accented language that you suspect is a combination of English and Creole. The television is on and food is displayed in several containers on the windowsill. You are looked at suspiciously when you enter and introduce yourself. The visitors do not offer to leave, but move back to make room for you near the patient's bed. Mrs. Thompson looks younger than her stated age, dressed in the hospital gown covered with a robe and her hair wrapped in a bright scarf. She smiles pleasantly and asks what you would like her to do. You answer, "Actually, this is all about what *you* want to do."

Questions as You Begin

Consider these questions as you begin developing this case:

- You know your best chance of having Mrs. Thompson accept any recommended changes is by incorporating them into her normal habits and routines, while respecting her culture and values. How can you learn about her cultural background?
- Should you ask her visitors to leave when you are working with her, ignore them, or include them in the process?

REFERENCES

1. Chan S. Chronic obstructive pulmonary disease and engagement in occupation. *Am J Occup Ther*. 2004;58: 408–415. doi:10.5014/ajot.58.4.408.

2. American Occupational Therapy Association. Occupational therapy practice framework: domain and process, 3rd ed. *Am J Occup Ther*. 2014;68:S1–S48. doi:10.5014/ajot.2014.682006.

Organ System Condition Cases

Organ system conditions are those conditions in which multiple organs or organ systems are affected, or there is a broad, systemic affect such as with diabetes. The cases presented here represent some of the more common conditions involving organ systems that an occupational therapist might treat; low vision, extensive burns, diabetes with renal failure and an amputation, and cancer with a mastectomy and lymphedema. In each case, the patient is struggling to regain their independence and the roles of student, caretaker or productive member of society, while coping with conditions causing weakness and pain, as well as stress and body image disturbances. You may encounter such conditions when the person comes for treatment at an inpatient setting, a specialty outpatient clinic, or through homecare as they try to adapt to a change in health status. Some changes may be permanent, and will require a "new normal" in your client's life, and other changes in health status may change daily or even hourly, testing our client's coping mechanisms.

As always, you will need a careful analysis of factors that either inhibit or support occupational performance, together with an openness to continually renegotiate intervention plans as necessary to assist your clients to achieve life satisfaction. Your skills to work on an interprofessional team will also be challenged as you think through these cases, due to the need for a variety of areas of expertise.

CASE

6.1

CLIENT: Lawrence Timmons, 72-year-old African American male

CONDITION: Low vision (open-angle glaucoma)

SETTING: Outpatient rehabilitation clinic

You work in a large medical center that has a variety of specialty clinics. The Director of the rehabilitation department has encouraged therapists to pursue continuing education in areas that will support patients from the clinics such as lymphedema, wound care, and low-vision services. You have worked at the center for about a year, and have particularly enjoyed working with clients with vision impairment. These clients generally benefit from a lot of creative problem solving for environmental modification, occupation-based interventions using adaptive equipment and techniques, and advocacy for needed services and resources.[1] You have been reading about the AOTA (American Occupational Therapy Association) specialty certification in low vision, and have decided to begin working toward this credential to further strengthen your skills with these clients.

When you see your schedule this morning, you are pleased to see that you have a new patient in the outpatient clinic today from the low-vision clinic. You decide to review the background information before you get too busy. You sign into the electronic medical record and search for the most recent information on Mr. Lawrence Timmons. You find demographic information and relevant health information from both his general practitioner, Dr. Azhar Tahir, and his ophthalmologist, Dr. Brandon Walker.

The demographic information reveals that Lawrence Timmons is a 72-year-old African American male who lives alone in a senior citizen apartment building. He is widowed, and lists his son Simon as his emergency contact. He is a retired plumber and he has Medicare insurance coverage, both Part A and Part B. He is a member of the African Methodist Episcopal Zion church. English is his primary language.

Mr. Timmons' medical history includes osteoarthritis of his hips and knees with a hip replacement 2 years ago, high blood pressure, and open-angle glaucoma. He underwent argon laser trabeculoplasty 1 year ago to help in the control of his glaucoma. His current medications include Naproxen for joint pain, Lisinopril for high blood pressure, and Acetazolamide for his glaucoma. Mr. Timmons' peripheral vision has been slowly deteriorating over the past 5 years, despite medication and laser surgery. A recent vision assessment by Dr. Walker determined that not only was his peripheral vision worse, but the acuity of his remaining central field vision had also shown a further significant decline. Dr. Walker referred Mr. Timmons for occupational therapy (OT) after learning of the impact his recent change in vision has had on his self-care and health maintenance. The notes indicate that Mr. Timmons has more difficulty preparing meals, which has led to a significant weight loss, he has experienced several falls at home, and according to his son he seldom leaves his apartment now.

You skimmed over a few older notes looking for additional information related to Mr. Timmons' support systems, interests, or performance issues. A social work note from a previous admission for his hip replacement surgery mentions that he was going to give up the family home at the urging of his children because of his declining health. He has a daughter, Denise, who lives about an hour away, and a son, Simon, who lives nearby with his family. The social work note mentioned that Mr. Timmons used to enjoy tending to his yard and doing home repairs. Anticipating the disruption from the change in living environment, he was referred to a Senior Center that operated out of the same senior housing complex so that he would remain socially active. It was not clear whether he had ever attended. You finished the chart and set your notes aside, feeling as though you almost knew Mr. Timmons after reading so much about him.

When it is time for Lawrence Timmons' appointment, you go out to meet him in the rehabilitation department's waiting area. A secretary gives you the chart she has prepared and points out Mr. Timmons. He is a small, elderly black man sitting with his hands clasped and his eyes closed. He has wrinkled khaki pants, and a black pullover shirt that looks too large for him. You notice his socks are mismatched, and his nails are long and in need of clipping. Beside him is a worried-looking middle-aged man who is probably his son, judging by the family resemblance. You approach him and ask, "Mr. Timmons?" The older man straightens up and lifts his head, looking in your direction. "I'm Lawrence Timmons," he says softly. You introduce yourself, making sure to let your smile reflect in your voice. When you ask him to accompany you to the back treatment area, both men stand. "Are you okay, Dad?" asks the younger man. "I'll be fine," says Mr. Timmons, "You can wait here." As you walk down the hall Mr. Timmons stays close to your side, taking short steps. Mr. Timmons says, "I hope you can help me. I think the doctor sent me here because he's given up. I just keep praying for the strength to deal with all this, but I'm not doing very well I'm afraid. The worst part is seeing how worried my kids are about me." You want to offer Mr. Timmons some comfort, but you know you shouldn't overpromise. "I have worked with several other clients with low vision," you tell him, "and usually when we put our heads together, you would be surprised at what we can come up with. But first I need to find out what kinds of things you need to do, and what you *want* to do."

Questions as You Begin

Consider these questions as you begin developing this case:

- What is Mr. Timmons' relationship with his son?
- Is that relationship changing because of the vision loss?
- What is Mr. Timmons' greatest fear? What is his *son's* greatest fear?
- Should you have invited his son to come back to the treatment area also?

CASE 6.2

CLIENT:	Amal Chaudhuri, 21-year-old Pakistani male
CONDITION:	Burns to hands and face
SETTING:	Hospital inpatient burn unit

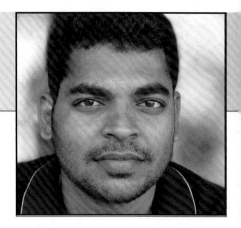

United Health Central is a large health organization made up of many different facilities. You work in the teaching hospital which houses most of the critical care units. You are a member of a large rehabilitation department that services a variety of these units. Today, you have received a new referral for a patient admitted 5 days ago to the burn unit. This special eight-bed unit takes on some of the most difficult burn cases in the region, and the employees who work together to serve these patients are proud of their reputation for having impressive outcomes. From the referral form, all you can tell is that the new patient is in bed 4 on the burn unit, his name is Amal Chaudhuri, and he is a 21-year-old male.

Signing into the online medical record system, you are able to access a lot of other information that lets you see him as a unique individual before you go in to make your first visit. From the demographic information you find out that Amal came to the United States 4 months ago on a study abroad program from Pakistan. He is a student at a local university studying business. He is listed as single, and his next of kin is listed as his father, who resides in Pakistan. He has one older sister who lives at home with his parents. His roommate and his dormitory director are also listed as local contacts. Religious affiliation is listed as Muslim. Primary language is listed as Urdu, but a note also indicates that he is fluent in English. Under insurance, the University is listed as providing coverage through private insurance.

The medical history and physical report indicate that Amal Chaudhuri was brought to the hospital by ambulance after an incident on campus during which students had started a bonfire. The police report given to the hospital stated that another student threw a flammable liquid on the fire and Amal received a "flash" burn to the front of his upper body as a result. He was conscious when he was brought in, and able to talk so he was not intubated. His respirations were good and he did not appear to have suffered from smoke inhalation. Once in the emergency department, he was directly admitted to the burn unit. His roommate came to the hospital with Amal, and provided some of the contact and background information. A central venous pressure (CVP) line was placed in his upper chest to provide and monitor fluid resuscitation and nutrients and administer intravenous morphine to control pain.

After the initial assessment of his condition it was determined that Amal had suffered burns to 30% of his body, including deep partial thickness burns to his hands, chest, and face with lesser burns to his right arm and neck. In the burn unit, the wounds were cleansed and debrided, occlusive dressings were applied to his hands and right arm, and his extremities were elevated to minimize the edema. His face and chest were treated with antibacterial cream, and then left open to let eschar form and dry. The plastic surgeon on the case decided that there was no need for skin grafting, and nursing and medical notes from the first 5 days indicate that Amal is healing well. Social work notes state that contact has been made with Amal's family in Pakistan, and his parents are making arrangements to come to the United States. Notes from nursing and social work indicate the patient is expressing some feelings of depression, with his greatest concern over his ability to use his hands again and return to school. He also expressed dismay that he is not able to practice his normal prayer activities.

Beginning today the occlusive dressings will be removed, and the patient is scheduled to start whirlpool three times per day for further debridement and joint mobilization. The eschar will be softened during the whirlpool with saline-soaked gauze to promote separation from the underlying healthy tissue that is forming. OT will start today with a primary goal to work on mobility of the hand and arm joints while the dressings are off in the whirlpool.

You call up to the floor and learn that Amal will have his next whirlpool at 2:00 PM. You arrive in the tank room several minutes early to introduce yourself. Amal seems anxious and tells you the pain during debridement was intense during his first whirlpool treatment earlier today, and he is dreading this one. You explain that you are there to gently work on his hands and arms, because you understand he wants to get them moving again in hopes of returning to school. Amal tells you he is into technology, and lives on the computer, his smartphone and loves gaming. Since his accident he says everything seems surreal, like his life has suddenly come to a screeching halt.

Questions as You Begin

Consider these questions as you begin developing this case:

- You know you will need to distract him while you are mobilizing his upper extremity joints. What should you talk about with him?
- If he is concerned about his prayer activities, then he likely has a strong faith. This may help him through this difficult time. How can you find out about traditional male Muslim practices?
- His movements will be restricted in this early phase of treatment. How can you incorporate some aspect of his faith into your practice?

CASE 6.3

CLIENT:	Ronald Knight, 60-year-old Caucasian male
CONDITION:	Type 1 diabetes with renal failure
SETTING:	Free-standing renal dialysis clinic

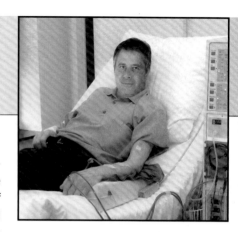

Wayne County Hospital provides not only traditional inpatient services, but also meets the healthcare needs of the region through a variety of outpatient services through both hospital-based and free-standing clinics. One of the busiest clinics is for outpatient dialysis, named The Turner Nephrology Clinic. The clients who fill the dialysis beds in this clinic typically have many chronic medical, personal/social, and economic needs. Staff from a variety of disciplines work together to coordinate care for these clients, with treatments being carried out during three 6-hour shifts. Often staff, clients and their families become close since the period of treatment may last months and sometimes years. When a client is fortunate enough to receive a kidney transplant, or is discharged to do home dialysis, everyone celebrates together. And when a client's transplant fails or a client passes away, they help one another grieve. Although some therapists find this work environment too intense and stressful, you can't imagine yourself working anyplace else. You are the only occupational therapist working with the dialysis clinic.

In the weekly team meeting on Monday, you heard that a new client was going to be starting on hemodialysis at the clinic this week. A medical file for the client is available on the electronic medical record system, and you find time after the meeting to review it. You start by looking at the demographic data that gives basic information about the patient. You see that Ronald Knight is a 60-year-old Caucasian male and a retired real estate agent. His wife Jenna is listed as next of kin. He lives in a large home in the suburbs of this small city. He receives social security disability and Medicare insurance coverage Part A and Part B. His religious affiliation is listed as Baptist.

Next, you turn to the social work section to get some more information related to personal context. From this section you learn that Mr. Knight has two children aged 20 and 24 years. Both children live in the area and see their parents frequently. Mrs. Knight works as a school psychologist, but has a flexible schedule so that she can be with Mr. Knight when she needs to. He retired young at 58 primarily due to worsening of his medical condition, and feeling that he was no longer able to provide the service he needed to for his customers. In his free time, Mr. Knight enjoys tinkering in his garage with vintage cars, home maintenance, and golf. He has a wide network of friends that he has developed over the years through his real estate contacts. He received a bachelor's degree in accounting at a local university. In spite of having lived with juvenile diabetes for most of his life, he has stayed relatively active until this past year due to his worsening condition.

Not surprisingly, the medical history section is very lengthy. As you scan through it, you note that Mr. Knight was diagnosed with type 1 diabetes at the age of 10. His insulin had been adjusted frequently over the ensuing years, as he and the doctors worked to keep his blood sugars regulated. In spite of going on an insulin pump at the age of 40, he developed diabetic retinopathy that affected his vision, and peripheral neuropathy causing reduced sensation and increased pain in his feet and hands. His ability to heal was compromised, as with most diabetics, and minor injuries from working with tools and gardening has twice led to serious infections in his left foot. Two years ago he had to give up driving due to his decreasing vision. A year ago he started to experience kidney failure.

Medication adjustments to manage his worsening condition had some positive results, but 2 weeks ago he entered the hospital in acute renal failure, suffering from nausea, shortness of breath, and muscle cramps. Temporary dialysis and additional medications were unsuccessful in regaining function in either kidney, and the decision was made to start him on regular hemodialysis. Since then, a venous catheter was placed in his chest to provide vascular access. Plans were made for an arteriovenous fistula to be developed later. Transportation arrangements have been made with a medical transport company to bring Mr. Knight to the dialysis clinic so that his wife will not have to provide transportation, since he will be coming to the center 3 days each week. Mr. Knight was discharged from the hospital yesterday with prescriptions for Lyrica for his peripheral neuropathy, Lantus and Humalog for diabetes, and Ferrous Sulphate for anemia.

On the intake form to the dialysis clinic, you note that Mr. Knight is scheduled to be on the afternoon shift, starting his treatment in chair 8 at 3:00 PM. His dialysis will take approximately 4 hours to complete, but is expected to take longer the first few times. You know the best time to work with your clients is about an hour after they have started dialysis, so you let the staff know that you plan to start your evaluation with him at 4:30 PM. You see Mr. Knight and his wife being welcomed by the staff just before 3:00 PM. He is wearing a pink shirt and seems to be in good spirits. You notice that his wife brought a notebook to write down information, and is looking more anxious than her husband. The dietitian meets with the couple around 4:00 PM and when she finishes you give Mr. Knight and his wife a few minutes alone before you go over and introduce yourself. Mrs. Knight says, "Everyone has been so nice, but I have to tell you it's a little overwhelming!" You smile and nod your head in understanding, and then add, "Part of my job, is to make sure you can still do the important things in your life–even with dialysis in the picture."

Questions as You Begin

Consider these questions as you begin developing this case:

- Is his wife's anxiety going to affect Mr. Knight?
- How can you address it without taking the focus off Mr. Knight?
- He, on the other hand, seems much more relaxed than most clients just starting dialysis. Could he be in denial? How should you proceed if he is?

CASE

6.4

CLIENT: Linda Randall, 58-year-old Caucasian female

CONDITION: Cancer with mastectomy and lymphedema

SETTING: Outpatient rehabilitation clinic

The outpatient center you work for, the Feldman Center, has developed a reputation for serving special populations, in addition to people with more typical musculoskeletal conditions. Some of these specialties include wound care, pregnant women with back pain, and lymphedema patients. You are an OT generalist, with no additional certifications in specialty areas, although you think you might be interested in becoming certified in lymphedema treatment someday. Because of your interest, you are especially pleased to receive a new referral to co-treat a client along with Diana, the physical therapist (PT) who has lymphedema certification.

The schedule today is very busy, and you have little time to talk with Diana other than to learn that your new client is "a really neat lady who is working hard to get her life back after cancer," and that the client will be there at 2:00 PM. This client has been coming for a week already to see the PT, so you know you can find additional information in the Center's chart. On the front sheet you learn that the client's name is Linda Randall. She is a 58-year-old Caucasian woman, with health insurance coverage through the federal Affordable Care Act. Under employment you notice it says "beautician." Religious affiliation is listed as Seventh Day Adventist. Her husband David is listed as the next of kin.

The referral form was filled out by Dr. Anwar, a local oncologist who has sent several of his patients to the Center for lymphedema treatments in the past. The diagnosis is given as, "lymphedema LUE status post radical mastectomy and radiation for breast cancer." Under the request section you see that she has written "OT/PT for post radical mastectomy with secondary lymphedema." There is also a copy of a recent medical history and physical report that had been sent over with the referral. From this you learn that Mrs. Randall had a modified radical mastectomy of her left breast for stage II breast cancer, followed by radiation. Although her cancer treatment was completed 4 months ago, she has recently developed lymphedema in her left upper extremity. You know that people are at higher risk of lymphedema after the lymph nodes have been blocked or disrupted, but you wonder if there was anything else that triggered the onset. There is no other significant surgery to note, but in the medical history you notice that she has hypothyroidism and has had several skin infections in her left arm and hand since her surgery.

Under the social history section it says that Mrs. Randall lives with her husband and two teenaged sons in a two-storey house in the center of town. She works in a beauty parlor and plans to return to work. She does not use tobacco and drinks alcohol only occasionally. Her husband was laid off 1 year ago from a construction firm and has been unable to find work. She has a lot of extended family in the area. She has a high school degree and is a licensed beautician. Under the family history section you notice that both her mother and an aunt have died from cancer. Her medications include Synthroid for her thyroid condition and Keflex for a skin infection.

Mrs. Randall arrives early for treatment. She is an attractive woman wearing a pretty sweater. You notice that she has poor posture, sitting with slouched shoulders in the waiting room. No one appears to have accompanied her. You notice that her left arm and hand are wrapped, and appear to be significantly larger than the right. You wait until Diana brings Mrs. Randall back to a treatment room before you join them. You are introduced to the client, and she asks you to please call her Linda. Diana explains that although she has been working with Linda to teach her how to wrap and manage her left arm, she is confident that you can help her regain her independence. Linda smiles and says, "That's why I like this place. I'm not just a diagnosis here, I'm a person." While Diana unwraps Linda's bandaged arm, you ask her to tell you about herself. "Well," she says, "until this all happened I worked about 50 or 60 hours a week, cooked up a storm for my boys and was on a bunch of committees at church. I was just starting to feel up to doing some things again after my surgery when this lymphedema started. But I have to get back to work soon because Dave hasn't been able to find work since he was laid off."

Once her arm is unwrapped you ask Linda to show you how her left hand is moving. She is able to move all joints, but cannot make a complete fist. Her wrist, elbow, and shoulder lack about 50% of normal mobility. "This is way better than it was a week ago," Diana tells you, "but I know we can make more progress."

Questions as You Begin

Consider these questions as you begin developing this case:

- With only partial mobility and weakness of her affected arm, what meaningful activities can you modify that will get her using her left arm again?
- It sounds like the family has limited financial resources. Should you avoid recommending any adaptive equipment because of this?
- What impact does Dave being off work have on Linda's roles and routines?
- You also wonder what impact Linda's mastectomy and lymphedema are having on their relationship.

REFERENCE

1. Warren M, Barstow E, eds. *Occupational Therapy Interventions for Adults with Low Vision*. Bethesda, MD: AOTA Press; 2011.

Mental Disorder Cases

The role of occupation in the treatment of mental illness is well documented since at least the late 1700s when the French physician Phillipe Pinel advocated the unshackling of the mentally ill, and the therapeutic use of occupation to aid in recovery.[1] The formal establishment of the occupational therapy movement in the United States in 1917 likewise grew out of the ongoing interest in the use of occupation to promote the humane treatment of the mentally ill. Since that time, public policy has shifted support for treatment of the mentally ill from inpatient to outpatient services, and most large inpatient psychiatric institutions were emptied and closed under the 1963 Community Mental Health Act.[2,3] However, the United States continues to struggle with identifying the best way to deliver services to people with chronic mental disorders.

The cases presented in this chapter represent a variety of settings, to reflect the complexity of the current service environment; short-term acute inpatient care, a behavioral health unit, an outpatient clinic, supportive housing with services, and a day-treatment program to support people with chronic mental disorders. The role of occupational therapy in these units is also evolving, and reflects our strength in assessing the global impact of symptomatology on performance, and grading client-centered interventions focused on physical, cognitive, psychological, and even spiritual development.

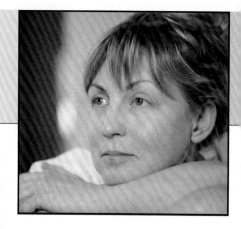

CASE

7.1

CLIENT: Melissa Clark, 53-year-old Caucasian female

CONDITION: Major depressive disorder with suicidal ideation

SETTING: Hospital inpatient mental health unit

You work at a regional medical center with both inpatient and outpatient mental health services. You split your time with 30 hours a week dedicated to the inpatient unit, and 10 hours a week in outpatient services. The inpatient unit has a 15-bed capacity with an average length of stay of 2 weeks. There are three different psychiatrists who admit to the unit. Other staff include a psychologist, a psychiatric social worker, nurses, and a recreation therapist. Patients are usually admitted to the unit either through the emergency department (ED) or direct admissions from the psychiatrists' offices or the county mental health clinic. The admissions are divided equally between voluntary admissions and involuntary commitments.

You provide treatment through therapeutic groups to individuals with a variety of mental disorders. However, the occupational therapy groups are divided not by diagnosis, but by severity of symptoms. Groups will vary by type of goals, and include organizational skills, communication or social interaction, self-care skills, instrumental activities of daily living (IADLs), and community reentry. You meet with each new patient individually at first to identify the patient's goals and collaborate on which therapeutic groups would be most beneficial.

At the morning briefing you learn that there was a new patient, Melissa Clark, admitted to the unit last night through the ED. The patient had been receiving treatment from one of the community psychiatrists, but had begun having suicidal thoughts yesterday and called her counselor's office. Her psychiatrist was out of town and Ms. Clark was advised by the counselor to have a family member take her to the closest ED. The social worker who saw her in the ED wrote that he had spoken with her brother by phone after receiving permission from the patient. The brother stated that he was very supportive of Melissa, and in fact she and his wife were quite close. Although he lives almost an hour away from his sister, she is welcome to stay with them if that would help her when she is discharged. The brother also said that he thought she was less depressed when she was working, and he hoped that she could return to work soon, as he and his wife both work, so there would be no one at home with her during the day if she were to stay with him.

You review the chart and find from the front sheet that Melissa Clark is 53 years old, is single, and has private insurance through her job as a legal secretary. Her brother is listed as next of kin and emergency contact. Her religious affiliation is noted to be Mormon. On the ED admission report you see that Ms. Clark is divorced and lives alone, and has one son in college. She has a brother and his family in the area, whom she called to bring her to the emergency room. She had been seeing a counselor weekly and a psychiatrist once a month for depression, which had started after her father died more than a year ago. Her depression had resulted in sleep disturbance, agitation, and inability to focus in addition to depressed mood. Medications had helped with sleep but had not been effective in dealing with the psychomotor symptoms or the low mood. She was taking Lexapro for depression and anxiety, and Ativan as needed for breakthrough anxiety and to promote sleep. She was unhappy with the side effects including weight gain, headaches, and lack of energy, and reported that she has not been taking either medication as prescribed, gradually decreasing her use over the last 2 months. The on-call psychiatrist did a screening in the emergency department and determined that Ms. Clark was severely depressed with specific suicidal ideation. She admitted to having similar suicidal thoughts before, which is why she originally sought treatment after her father's death. The psychiatrist recommended admission to the inpatient psychiatric unit, and Ms. Clark agreed to a voluntary admission. No medications were prescribed by the emergency department's on-call psychiatrist. The intake nurse charted that the patient was concerned about having no sleeping medications.

The nursing team leader had reported at the meeting that the patient had not reached the unit from the emergency department until two o'clock this morning, and had been allowed to sleep past the usual 7:00 AM medication pass since she was on no medications yet. Doctor Zhan stated he would interview Ms. Clark after the team meeting, and discuss his plans to discontinue her last prescribed psychotropic medications and start her on Cymbalta the next morning if the laboratory results show that her body is clear of the previous medications. Although nursing reported that she was demonstrating some tremors and difficulty concentrating at admission, the psychiatrist encouraged you to have the new patient attend one of the therapeutic groups today, and observe her for symptoms of medication withdrawal, particularly from Lexapro.

Finishing your review of the chart, you decide to see if Melissa is in the common room. Since you are familiar with all of the other patients, you spot her quickly sitting alone at one of the tables. She is a Caucasian woman of medium build, with short medium blonde hair. She has her head down on her arms and her eyes are closed. When you approach and call her name, she lifts her head slowly and looks at you. You notice she looks anxious, and her hands are shaking. But when you smile and introduce yourself, asking if you can speak with her she nods her head. "I'd like to have you come to one of my groups today," you tell her. "The doctor thinks it would be good for you, and I do as well." "What would I have to do?" she asks slowly. You tell her it depends on which group she attends, which is why you want to talk to her, to understand her better. "Everyone here is working on different goals, so that things will be better when they are discharged. Can you tell me how your depression has affected you at work and at home?" There is a long pause before she answers. "I'm just so down all the time." She says. "It's too hard. Everything is overwhelming." When you ask her what she used to enjoy doing in her free time she tells you scrap booking and trying new recipes. You ask her what the most difficult thing at home is and she replies, "Being alone. I'm too tired to keep the house up. I can't face going back there."

Questions as You Begin

Consider these questions as you begin developing this case:

- Clearly her depression has been affecting all aspects of Melissa's life. Managing the side effects of the medications could be a key to helping her stay on them long term. Which of the groups would be best to support her ability to work on coping with the common side effects?
- Should you ask her about her suicidal ideation directly when you're working with her, or leave that to the psychiatrist?

CASE

7.2

CLIENT: Roberto Alvarez, 22-year-old Hispanic
                 male

CONDITION: Bipolar disorder with manic episode

SETTING: Mental health day treatment program

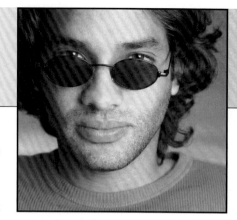

The county mental health clinic has a variety of services, and works cooperatively with an integrated program of services throughout the region. As an occupational therapist, you work primarily at the mental health day treatment and outpatient program. The program is located in an old elementary school building that the county purchased several years ago and refurbished. Although the building has typical problems with the mechanical systems and roof, many of the features are ideal for your program, including the gymnasium, a small auditorium, and a central courtyard for private outdoor space and gardening. Occupational therapy is a key part of the program, helping clients manage their conditions, develop life skills, and make progress toward meaningful vocational and avocational goals. You work with an interesting group of people with a variety of chronic mental disorders. Most clients will remain with the program for several years. Although it is not unusual for a client to experience an episode of increased symptoms and require short-term hospitalization, the program has a solid track record of reducing the need for inpatient treatment by helping clients live successfully in the community with support.

Tomorrow a new client will be starting your program. Roberto Alvarez was referred by the outpatient mental health counseling program. You sit down to review what information was sent over with the referral to get a better understanding of Mr. Alvarez. On the front sheet of the information you received from the outpatient program, you see that he is 22 years old and is diagnosed with bipolar disorder, type I. His next of kin is listed as his father. There is no employer listed. Spanish is listed under the heading: primary language. Mr. Alvarez has Medicaid listed for his insurance. The medical history and physical report do not show anything remarkable, other than surgery following a knife fight, where Mr. Alvarez was knifed in his abdomen, and a fractured leg from a fall from a balcony. When you read the counselor's latest progress note, you started to get a better understanding of the chaotic life of Roberto Alvarez. This client was diagnosed at 15 with bipolar disorder, after several episodes of manic behavior that landed him in trouble at school and with the authorities, which were then followed by periods sometimes lasting several months when he was so depressed he wouldn't leave his bed for days. After one of these long spells of depression his father took him into the emergency room. He was placed on an antidepressant and within days was in a severe state of mania with agitation, delusions of grandeur, and pressured speech. It was during this episode when he jumped from a balcony and fractured his leg. His diagnosis was then determined to be manic depression and a mood stabilizer was then used with better results. He dropped out of school at 16 in spite of being a good student, even with multiple absences. After that he intermittently received treatment, and went on and off of psychotropic medications that he was prescribed. At 17, he was committed to a facility for juvenile delinquents after his arrest for stealing a computer.

While in the facility, he obtained his General Education Degree (GED) for high school, and was stable, taking his medication consistently. He was released at age 18 and returned home to live with his father, stepmother, and two younger half-siblings.

Roberto Alvarez had worked several part-time and temporary jobs, but had a pattern of going off his medication and becoming impulsive and stubborn, and doing something that would lead to the loss of another job. His father had reached a point where he told his son he had to leave because he was a bad influence on his brother and sister. Alvarez had reportedly "couch surfed," living with various friends and working odd jobs for about 6 months. About 4 months ago he promised his father he would go to counseling and stay on his medication, and his father had allowed him to return home. He had been consistent in attending counseling, developing a good relationship with one of the counselors, and joining a support group. Although he had experienced one bout of depression since starting counseling, he was fairly stable on a combination of Olanzapine (Zyprexa) and Zoloft. The counselor was concerned, however, because he had gotten in a fight with his stepmother and left home, and hadn't taken his medications for several days last week. When he came to his therapy appointment last week, he was demonstrating agitation and pressured speech, and said he wasn't sure he needed the medicine because it made him feel "slow." The counselor talked with him about the consequences of not taking the medication, and he voiced understanding. When she suggested that he try attending the day treatment program he expressed reservations, saying that it was "probably for psychos," and stating that he would prefer to have a job so that he could get his own apartment. The counselor's assessment at the end of last week was that the client was possibly entering a manic phase, and being able to help him stay on his medications and in a routine would be critical. She is not sure he will show up at the day treatment program, but the patient's father has promised to bring him. In one of the counselor's notes you see that he had mentioned that his leisure interests are playing computer games and "building things."

The next day you watch for your new client as people are arriving. You notice Roberto right away–a thin, young man with a red shirt and glasses. He is looking around, carefully watching everyone and hanging back. You notice that he shifts from foot to foot, and keeps putting his hands in and out of his pockets. You approach him with a smile and introduce yourself. He tells you to call him "Robert" and gets right to his concerns. "So what is this place, anyway?" he asks.

Questions as You Begin

Consider these questions as you begin developing this case:

- Roberto seems to have maintained a positive, though tenuous relationship with his father. Can you use that to motivate him to participate in the program?
- Or would it be better to motivate him with the vocational skills development aspect of the program?
- You are concerned that his attitude that the other clients are "psychos" may not only keep him from participating, but it is insulting and unfair to the other clients. At the same time, you can't tell Roberto about the other clients' conditions. How should you handle this?

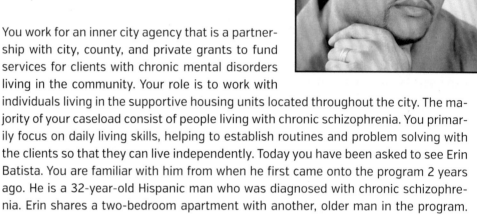

CASE 7.3

CLIENT:	Erin Batista, 32-year-old Hispanic male
CONDITION:	Paranoid schizophrenia with psychosis
SETTING:	Home program to help people with chronic mental health issues

You work for an inner city agency that is a partner-ship with city, county, and private grants to fund services for clients with chronic mental disorders living in the community. Your role is to work with individuals living in the supportive housing units located throughout the city. The majority of your caseload consist of people living with chronic schizophrenia. You primarily focus on daily living skills, helping to establish routines and problem solving with the clients so that they can live independently. Today you have been asked to see Erin Batista. You are familiar with him from when he first came onto the program 2 years ago. He is a 32-year-old Hispanic man who was diagnosed with chronic schizophrenia. Erin shares a two-bedroom apartment with another, older man in the program. Both men attended a day-treatment program 5 days a week, and Erin has been able to get some supervised employment through the program, cleaning office buildings two nights a week. Once his routine was established and he was doing well, you had discontinued him from your regular services.

One of the psychiatric social workers sent you a message asking you to put him back on your service again. She was concerned about him because he had stopped attending the work program, was reportedly participating less at day treatment, and had shown up for a session with her looking very disheveled last week, and she suspected his auditory hallucinations were worse because of his decreased concentration. You had a chance yesterday to take a look at his records. You see that he is taking an atypical antipsychotic medication called Risperidone. In the past, when he has experienced increased symptoms he becomes quite suspicious of others, and has auditory hallucinations telling him to hurt himself. It is not certain if he is ever free of the hallucinations, but when he is stable, Erin is able to concentrate quite well, and maintain healthy daily living skills to care for himself and his apartment, prepare simple meals, and use public transportation. Difficult areas for him have always been dealing with inconsistency in rules and routines, maintaining personal relationships, and problem solving when feeling stressed. He enjoys reading, researching information online, and writing poetry.

When you called Erin yesterday evening to tell him that you wanted to visit today after he returned from his program, he was quite subdued. He did finally admit he remembered you from before, but he seemed concerned about why you wanted to visit. You explained that his counselor was concerned about him and wanted you to visit to see if there was anything you could do to help him. He seemed satisfied with this and agreed to your visit.

When you walk up the hall toward his door, you see Erin peering out. He immediately closes the door when he sees you. When you knock he doesn't answer. After calling his name and telling him who you are the door is finally opened. The room is dark and you see empty cans and dishes scattered about. Among them you notice some empty pill containers. You tell Erin, "I'm glad to see you. I enjoyed helping you before, and I'd like to help you again if that's okay. Why don't you tell me what's been going on lately?"

Questions as You Begin

Consider these questions as you begin developing this case:

- How should you respond to evidence of auditory hallucinations while you are meeting with Mr. Batista?
- It appears that there are no medications or food in the apartment, but he is afraid to go to the store. His safety is at risk if you cannot see that he has access to food and medications within a short period of time. How should you handle this?

CASE

7.4

CLIENT:	Mary Anne Warren, 34-year-old Caucasian female
CONDITION:	Posttraumatic stress disorder with alcohol abuse
SETTING:	Inpatient behavioral health program

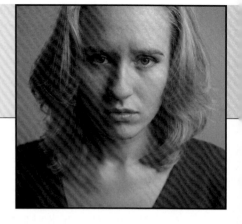

You work with an inpatient behavioral health program that treats people with alcohol and other drug addictions, with or without mental disorders. You have learned that sometimes your clients have primary mental disorders that they are "self-treating" with alcohol and drugs, and other people have primary addiction problems that are aggravating underlying mental disorders. The philosophy of the program is that addiction is an illness that affects the central nervous system. The maladaptive behavior that is a symptom of the disorder can be managed through a cognitive–behavioral treatment approach. Clients receive both individual and group therapy to understand their condition, identify unhealthy thought patterns, and work on developing coping skills and self-esteem. Medication is used when needed to address depression, anxiety, or other mental disorders, but pain medication and sleeping medication are not prescribed to past narcotic users. Clients are admitted to the program after completing withdrawal in an acute care setting, and after symptoms of existing mental disorders have been stabilized. This program is a 28-day residential program. About half of the clients are referred from hospitals or acute mental health settings, and the other half are court ordered into treatment, often as an alternative for jail.

You have a new admission today named Mary Anne Warren. You will be meeting her in the morning group after breakfast, so you take a few minutes to gather some background information from the medical chart. You see from the face sheet that she is 34 and has insurance through the federal Affordable Care Act. A female friend is listed as the emergency contact. The intake counselor was able to get quite a complete history leading up to her admission to the program. Mary Anne grew up in a troubled home with a lot of dysfunction. When she was 15, she witnessed the murder of her older brother by her stepfather. In the years that followed, she tried to put her past behind her, leaving home and joining college, making new friends, and seldom having contact with her family. She completed a Bachelor's degree in marketing and found part-time work with a bookstore. Now she is 34 and told the counselor that she is haunted by her past. She has nightmares about her brother and stepfather. She feels anxious all the time, becoming increasingly preoccupied that something terrible is about to happen to her. She recently broke off a relationship with a boyfriend, only saying, "I can't be with him anymore, I can't trust him."

Several girlfriends had tried to help her, but she says she can't talk to them and admits she has closed herself off more and more. She has stopped going out with friends, saying it makes her too nervous to be around a lot of people, especially strangers. She used to enjoy trying new restaurants and going to movies, but has not gone out in a long time because she becomes anxious in new places. She works part time as a supervisor at a bookstore, and her boss told her that he is not happy with her performance because she is not making decisions, and seldom wants to be out with customers, preferring to stay in the office and work on paperwork. What her friends and boss did not know is that for the past 2 years she has been drinking every night at home, secretly hoping it will block out the night terrors and the anxiety she feels. And to a certain extent, it did work, because she would eventually pass out and sleep. She worked afternoons and evenings at the store, which gave her time to pull herself back together in the mornings so people wouldn't know. Lately she stops at the liquor store every few nights on her way home from work, and she has progressively been drinking more and stronger liquor. It all became unraveled when a friend had decided to stop in on a whim to check on her, and was appalled to find her almost unconscious, not making sense and talking about how someone was going to kill her.

The friend called 911 and Mary Anne was taken to a local emergency room where she was assessed by a medical intern and the on-call psychiatrist. She was admitted first to the intensive care unit for 3 days while she went through alcohol withdrawal, then to the acute inpatient mental health clinic on a voluntary commitment for 2 weeks where she was diagnosed with posttraumatic stress disorder (PTSD). She was stabilized on Nardil and Ativan, and began opening up with the staff on the unit and in therapy. The staff at the acute inpatient program recommended that Mary Anne complete additional treatment through the behavioral health program to further address her alcohol addiction as well as her PTSD and anxiety.

After you finish your review of the chart you are interested to meet your new client. You join the psychiatric social worker and one of the nurses in the day room for the morning meeting. The morning group is fairly unstructured, but includes introductions of anyone who is new, and a review of the day's activities. Everyone, including the staff, then share briefly one personal behavioral goal they are going to work on that day. You notice Mary Anne right away. She looks tired, pale, and anxious, fidgeting in her seat. She quietly moves to another seat when a male client takes one next to her. She doesn't say anything other than her first name when she is asked to introduce herself. She keeps her head down and does not make eye contact with anyone.

Questions as You Begin

Consider these questions as you begin developing this case:

- Mary Anne does not trust men, and there are predominantly male staff and typically far more men than women clients in the program. How can you be sensitive to her fears while helping her cope with interacting with men?
- Vocational rehabilitation is not part of your program. Still, the fact that she has a job is a strength. How should you help Mary Anne with work reentry, or should you?

REFERENCES

1. Wilcock AA. *Occupation for Health: A Journey from Self Health to Prescription*. London: College of Occupational Therapists; 2001.
2. Ray CG, Finley JK. Did CMHCs fail or succeed? Analysis of the expectations and outcomes of the community mental health movement. *Admin Policy Ment Health.* 1994;21(4):283–284.
3. Accordino MP, Porter DF, Morse T. Deinstitutionalization of persons with severe mental illness: context and consequences. *J Rehabil.* 2001;67(2):16–21.

Interprofessional Cases

In 2014, the American Occupational Therapy Association (AOTA) published several important papers clarifying the role of occupational therapists on interprofessional care teams. The AOTA's Position Paper, *The role of occupational therapy in primary care*[1] noted that OT (occupational therapy) practitioners are well prepared to contribute to interprofessional care teams. Our focus on function with everyday life skills by addressing ADLs (activities of daily living) and IADLs (instrumental activities of daily living) performance, as well as our knowledge of the impact that habits and routines have on individuals' health and wellness, will provide a valuable contribution to primary care teams.

A continuing education article, *Occupational therapy in primary care: an emerging area of practice*,[2] concluded that OT practitioners need to both continue efforts to educate physicians, other disciplines, and politicians about the value of OT, and participate in the early formation of new models of practice that are being developed in response to healthcare reform to ensure that OTs are included in developing interprofessional care teams.

Such multidisciplinary health teams are not new to health care. Precursors to the emerging primary care teams were the hospital discharge planning committees and mental health interdisciplinary teams, to name only a few. The focus, however, in the newer interprofessional teams has distinct differences. As early as 1972, Pelligrino described this difference as each member of the team not only contributing their discipline's unique knowledge and skills, but also integrating their perspective with other disciplines to create an individualized approach to client's health challenges.[3] The interprofessional team takes a much longer view, crossing the boundaries of the healthcare practice settings and following clients over the course of chronic health problems, putting an equal or even greater emphasis on illness prevention and wellness than illness intervention and management. Emerging payment systems support long-term relationships between clients and their primary care team, with bundled payments and other reimbursement models that incentivize management of chronic disease in a coordinated manner that meets quality outcome standards and ultimately lowers the cost of health care.[4]

The need to prepare entry-level occupational therapy and therapy assistant students for interprofessional collaborative practice has been underscored by the Accreditation Council for Occupational Therapy Education (ACOTE) in their 2013 Standards and Interpretive Guide,[5] standard B.5.21. The emphasis of this new standard is to prepare students to work constructively on interprofessional teams by being able to effectively communicate with and understand the roles of other disciplines in carrying out a comprehensive intervention plan.

Using cases to engage students of different professions in interactive learning is an ideal way to meet the goal of interprofessional education. The cases that follow represent different practice settings, but would reasonably benefit from a variety of professional interventions. The key to using these cases will be to learn about, from, and with other disciplines to coordinate your care with a true interprofessional approach.

The first case represents the challenges of a more traditional inpatient discharge coordination team, working together to prepare client-centered and safe discharges for several clients over the course of a busy day. The second case represents a challenging home hospice setting that brings together a variety of disciplines to meet a client and her family's complex end-of-life needs. In the third case, an interprofessional team collaborates to develop services for the homeless population, creating a homeless outreach program in an urban area.

The final case represents a client struggling to manage a chronic disease, diabetes, which has led to severe complications and multiple inpatient admissions. A specialty primary care clinic with an interprofessional team approach will work to help him manage his health challenges and maintain quality of life, while minimizing the need for inpatient care.

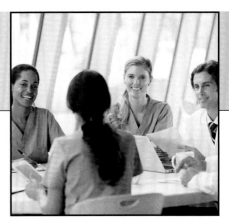

CASE

8.1

SITUATION: A day in the life of a busy discharge coordination team

CONDITION: Varied

SETTING: Hospital inpatient setting

The discharge coordination team that you are a member of meets every morning in a busy medical center. Representatives on the team come from a variety of departments and functions throughout the center, but work collaboratively to ensure that the discharges of all patients are safe and efficient, and in concert with patient's expectations. In the old days, employees would just give a status report on patients, and then nursing and social work staff would work with physicians to finish a discharge. But the entire process was redesigned about a year ago to make quality improvements. Patient satisfaction surveys reflected low ratings for discharge planning. There were too many patients returning to the hospital for follow-up care after discharge. And even though no one wanted to admit it, there were too many mistakes being made: missed referrals, equipment and supplies not delivered to patient's home before discharge, and lack of adequate patient education. After charging individual departments with making changes, it was finally decided that a more integrated approach was needed.

Now, key departments had dedicated staff that received training in group process and communication. A hospitalist or nurse practitioner chaired the meeting, although there had been discussion about rotating the leadership between disciplines. One of the discharge planning coordinators (usually with background in nursing or social work) brought the names of patients who were about to be discharged or nearing the end of their length of stay. Social workers were requested to tell patients about the purpose of the upcoming meeting and interview them or their families about discharge preferences, needs, and concerns prior to the meeting. Patients or a family member were welcome to attend the meeting during the pertinent discussion if they desired. Each team member made sure that they were up to speed on the status of all patients being seen by their department. What made this meeting different was how the team members collaborated to come up with the best solution as a whole, from the perspective of the patient and their healthcare needs alone. It was tough sometimes, when one of the members thought the patient would benefit from something, particularly a service they cared about strongly, and other members disagreed; or when members disagreed on a patient's abilities or safety needs. Ultimately, the team had to come together behind a solid plan that the patient and his or her family could buy into. Communication, compromise, and a willingness to question each other, as well as making the patient the focus were usually the keys to success. On any given day, the team might review 15 patients in the morning meeting, with between 3 and 5 of them needing significant team planning.

The results had been positive over the past year since the meetings were redesigned. Outcome measures on patient satisfaction, readmissions within 2 weeks of discharge, and errors related to the discharge process were all improved. Two people had requested to step down from the team due to team conflict that they were uncomfortable with, and one of the hospitalists had been discouraged from leading the team, due to poor team leadership and communication skills.

Today's schedule looks pretty typical. When the discharge planner hands out the list of patients, there are three highlighted, indicating they need significant discussion. One of them, Marge Francis, has a note next to it that the patient wanted to attend the meeting. The team moves efficiently through the first group of patients who are nearing discharge in a few days, but have no significant concerns indicated by any of the disciplines. Rehabilitation is requested to pick up one of the patients that is not on their service, due to concerns of deconditioning and a frail spouse at home. The rehabilitation representative at the meeting noted that their department was short staffed, but agreed the situation was a safety concern and assured the team that the patient would be picked up. A social work representative expressed concern about a woman admitted for a broken jaw and collapsed lung, suspected to be a victim of domestic abuse, but unwilling to discuss it. The team brainstormed potential services that could be brought in while the patient was still in the hospital to see if she could be helped, but several team members noted that the patient's rights to refuse any service, and confidentiality when talking to outside agencies had to be carefully considered.

The three cases that were in need of significant planning are each described below. Your interprofessional team has 20 to 30 minutes to discuss and develop a transition plan for each patient. All relevant disciplines' perspectives must be considered, and the plan must meet the client's needs and preferences. The discharge must be considered safe by all disciplines involved in the meeting.

Case 1: Bernard Giuseppe

Bernard Giuseppe is a 78-year-old Caucasian male who was admitted through the emergency department after being brought in by an ambulance from a family care home in a rural area. He had a note in his pocket that said, "We cannot take him back here. He needs too much care." The ambulance crew had reported that they were called to the home because the man had fallen and the staff were unable to get him up. X-rays in the emergency department revealed a fracture at the neck of the left femur. The emergency department staff were unsuccessful in contacting the family care home or in locating any family members, and the patient was disoriented in all three spheres. The dietary representative reported that the patient was well below ideal body weight and had no teeth and no dentures. The hospitalist leading the group expressed concern that Mr. Giuseppe was not a good candidate for hip surgery, due to his mental state and some cardiac and electrolyte issues that were indicated by the lab results. He had contacted an orthopedic surgeon to see whether at least a pinning should be tried to stabilize the fracture and reduce pain. The social work representative reported that they had been successful in contacting the family care home this morning, but information so far had not resulted in identifying any relatives. The staff at the home reported that Mr. Giuseppe was not allergic to anything, and usually didn't take any medication except an occasional laxative. They reported that he spoke broken English, and that Italian was his primary language.

The home claimed they were not the patient's guardian, and that he had always paid for their services from his Social Security checks, which came to him through mail to the home. They insisted that he could not return to the home because they were not equipped to handle someone who needed help ambulating or transferring. Nursing staff remarked that the patient had been combative with care at first, needing a great deal of reassurance before allowing the staff to insert intravenous hydration and a catheter to monitor fluids. He ate a pureed diet well this morning, feeding himself with setup and minimal assistance. He would not allow staff to feed him, even though he struggled with the utensils. He had several open areas on his extremities and back that were not pressure areas, and might have been from falls that had not healed well. His lungs were clear; however, he was slightly dehydrated. He did appear to have some pain in his injured leg, and was restless with the full leg abduction wedge in place, but had slept fairly well after receiving ibuprofen 200 mg tabs (dosage, 2 for pain). The nursing staff wanted to give him something stronger for pain, but the physician was concerned with making the dementia worse. In hopes of clearing his mental status, Mr. Giuseppe was started on Namenda for confusion at 10 mg twice per day. The rehabilitation representative stated that they were awaiting physician referral and had not yet performed an assessment. Several team members agreed with the rehabilitation service's request for a referral to begin bedside therapy even before a decision was made for surgery, in order to avoid deconditioning and to assist with assessing cognitive status and communication abilities, as well as to begin working with him on simple ADLs.

The social worker on the team wondered if the client had been abused at the home, and if she should call Adult Protective Services. Two other members of the team felt she was overreacting and did not have any evidence to support this. The rehabilitation representative felt no decisions about discharge could be made until it was determined if there was any chance Mr. Giuseppe was going to be able to weight-bear again. The discussion and planning continued as a preliminary discharge plan was developed to meet the patient's needs.

Case 2: Carlos Menendez

Carlos Menendez is an 18-year-old Hispanic male admitted through the emergency department 2 days ago after being brought in by friends with a gunshot wound to his right upper arm that occurred during a fight. On admission, he was unconscious and needed blood transfusions, followed by surgery to clean and close the wound. It was too early to tell if there would be any permanent loss of function in his right, dominant arm and hand, but there did not appear to be any significant nerve damage, according to the surgeon who operated. The police had been notified as per policy about the gunshot wound. Two detectives came to speak with the patient once he was alert after surgery.

Once awake, Carlos had insisted that he had no relationship with either of his parents, and as he was 18 he did not want them to be called. Although Carlos stated that he could sign for his own treatment, the attending physician admitted he felt uncomfortable treating him further without a parent's agreement. When asked about finances or insurance, Carlos stated that he only worked occasionally with a friend doing house painting and had no health insurance, and he would need help applying for aid. Two young males came to visit him in his room and had to be asked to leave when an argument broke out between them and the patient. Carlos gave his girlfriend's house as his permanent address, but when a social worker contacted the home, he was told that Carlos only slept there sometimes, and the woman Carlos had identified as his girlfriend stated it was not his permanent home address. The woman offered that Carlos was sometimes mixed up in gang activity, but said she did not know what had led to the shooting incident.

When this information was shared with the patient, he stated his girlfriend was just mad at him because of the fight, but she would "settle down" and he was sure he could go back there after discharge. The social worker did not feel this was a viable option due to the girlfriend's reluctance on the phone. Carlos shared that he had dropped out of school the year before, when he was a senior. A drug screen showed low levels of cocaine and marijuana in his system. The dietitian noted that Carlos was poorly nourished and had a poor appetite. He was on 10 mg intramuscular morphine every 4 hours for pain; however, the nursing staff wanted to discuss a patient-controlled analgesia machine with morphine to see if his pain would be better controlled.

An initial rehabilitation screening was done yesterday; the report indicated that there was some numbness in his right forearm as well as weakness in finger and wrist extension, but movement of all digits was present. The patient claimed to be in a great deal of pain, demanding pain medication throughout the screening. The rehabilitation representative questioned giving the patient control of the pain medication if there was a possible history of drug abuse. An animated discussion followed as the team worked through the case to prepare a preliminary discharge plan.

Case 3: Marge Francis

Marge Francis was brought to the meeting room by the nurse. She was wearing a hospital gown and had an intravenous pole with her. A catheter bag could be seen at the side of the wheelchair. She was receiving oxygen from a portable tank. She looks tired, but alert. The nurse introduced Mrs. Francis to the group and offered to share some of the background, and the patient nodded her head in agreement. The nurse proceeded, stating that Marge Francis is a 48-year-old African American woman admitted to the hospital with intractable pain from lung cancer. Although she had been through both chemotherapy and radiation therapy over the past 3 years, she was now suffering from metastases and was in the late stages of the disease. She also had a history of schizophrenia, which had been sporadically treated. On admission, Mrs. Francis stated that she was currently divorced, but that she had been married three times and that she has nine children. Mrs. Francis was accompanied to the hospital by her daughter, Luanne, who stated that she was 18. Luanne revealed that there were four more children at home besides herself, between the ages of 4 and 14 years.

The social worker then took over, reminding Mrs. Francis of their meeting on the previous day. She stated that she was concerned about supervision of the younger children while Mrs. Francis was in the hospital, and stated that Luanne had mentioned a grandmother who would occasionally come to help out, when her mother had to go to the hospital, but this did not seem as though it had been arranged.

Mrs. Francis shared that she had just recently moved her family to the area to be closer to her mother, but had not yet gotten the children settled into school. There were other extended relatives in the area, but the patient stated that she had not been close to any of them for many years. She had moved her children back to the area in hopes that relatives would take them in "when the time came."

The physician then asked Mrs. Francis to tell them about her current health problems. Mrs. Francis stated that she had been a chronic smoker since a young age, and even after she was first diagnosed with lung cancer she had been unable to stop smoking. She did not want to pursue any more treatment for her condition, stating "They did what they could." She would not say much about her mental health diagnosis, other than that she had been on Risperdal 2 mg twice a day for her "nerves" for many years. When asked how she felt when she was off the medication, she just said "You don't want to know." The physician had placed her on Roxanol for the pain, administered 1 mL (20 mg) every 4 hours as needed, and he asked how that was working.

The nurse stated that Mrs. Francis seemed to like the ease of taking the drops of medication and the patient agreed that it worked quickly and took care of most of the pain. The dietitian stated that Mrs. Francis loved ice cream and sweets, but would eat little else from her trays. Mrs. Francis did not respond to this comment.

The social worker asked the team what they thought of the idea of trying to get all of the children and maybe even the grandmother in for a meeting. Although several members of the team thought that would be helpful to meet with the family, the physician stated she thought it sounded like chaos, and as long as Mrs. Francis could make her own decisions they could just work with her.

Mrs. Francis seemed rather aloof during this discussion, but did not encourage a meeting with her children and mother. When asked if she had a living will or healthcare agent, Mrs. Francis answered no, but that her mother could do that if she needed to designate someone. The social worker said that she would help her with that, and offered to meet with both the patient and her mother to talk about how the children were to be cared for. The physician suggested that she would try to track down Mrs. Francis' previous oncologist to understand what her course of treatment had been, although the patient did not seem to think that this was important. The rehabilitation staff stated that they had received a referral but were not sure how they could best help Mrs. Francis. She then told them that she wanted to get strong enough to go home, and that she wanted to be able to die at home, not in the hospital. The rehabilitation representative then said "We can definitely help you work on that. Can you tell us some more about your home and what you need to be able to do in order to go back there?" Mrs. Francis left soon after, and the group proceeded to develop a plan to meet their patient's wishes and healthcare needs.

Questions as You Begin

Consider these questions as you begin:

- What impact does having the patient in attendance have on the meeting dynamics?
- How would you rate your team skills? Would you be effective on a team like this?
- What can you do to strengthen your interprofessional skills?

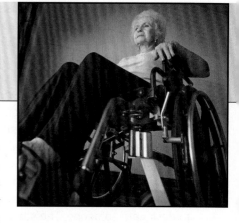

CASE 8.2

CLIENT:	Lynnette Wise, 60-year-old Caucasian female
CONDITION:	Amyotrophic lateral sclerosis
SETTING:	Home hospice program

You work for a regional hospice program that provides services by sending their trained staff into hospitals, skilled nursing facilities, and private homes to work with clients who come onto your program. Your agency has received a referral for a 60-year-old woman with amyotrophic lateral sclerosis (ALS) who is living at home with her husband and teenaged son. One of the hallmarks of your program is how well the different disciplines of the team coordinate and collaborate, not only with each other, but with the healthcare staff at the various agencies that are also providing ongoing care for the client.

Your agency has practitioners from a variety of disciplines including nurses; social workers; physical, occupational, and speech therapists; pharmacists; pastoral care; psychologists; and dietitians. All staff have additional training in end-of-life care. Occasionally, additional staff are added to the team on a consulting basis as needed for specific cases.

The team from your agency is meeting this morning to discuss Mrs. Wise and determine what services she needs, and how best to deliver those. At the meeting, you hear the following information from the intake coordinator: Two years ago, Lynette Wise was working as a phlebotomist at a local hospital when she began to notice that she was having difficulty with her fine motor skills. Things she had previously done without thinking were suddenly much more difficult. She also noticed some weakness in her legs, and she had a few unexplained falls. A visit to her doctor did not produce a diagnosis, so she had been sent to a neurologist. Although he initially suspected multiple sclerosis (MS), she did not have any eye involvement, which is often an early sign of MS or the typical pattern of episodes. A series of additional tests finally led to the diagnosis of ALS. She had already retired by the time she received the diagnosis. Her husband is a retired carpenter and spends much of his day "puttering" in a home workshop. He doesn't say much, but he is adamant about doing whatever is needed to keep her at home.

Their home is a single-storey home with a finished basement that he built himself. Since his wife became ill, he has built a ramp on the front of the house, a new addition for a master bedroom, a wheelchair accessible bathroom, and a beautiful deck that faces the hill behind their house. They have a daughter who lives nearby with two grandchildren. Although their daughter works as a schoolteacher, she comes over every evening and cooks, and both families eat dinner together.

Mrs. Wise is worried about the physical, psychological, and financial burden that she will be on her husband. When she was asked about her wishes, she told the staff she also wants to stay home, and not go back to the hospital if at all possible. Her symptoms right now are quadriparesis, decreased coordination with her hands, fatigue, muscle spasms with some nerve pain, and tremors. She has not had any swallowing difficulties so far, but she knows that is inevitable. She has just recently lost her ability to control her bladder, which really bothers her. Her medications right now are Gabapentin 300 mg twice a day for nerve pain, Ativan 2 mg twice a day for anxiety, and Ditropan 5 mg daily for bladder spasms. There is a housekeeper who comes in once a week to do some light housework and the laundry. A private aide has been coming in three times a week to help Mrs. Wise bathe. Her favorite pastimes are sitting on the back deck to watch her grandchildren play, using the computer, going to church, and watching television. She knows that her doctor has given her less than 6 months to live. She has declined to be involved in any clinical trials. She says that she just wants to be able to be with her family as much as possible, while not being a burden on them. She has Medicare Part A and Part B for health insurance coverage.

Questions as You Begin

Consider these questions as you begin developing this case:

- In what way is the church a possible resource for this family, to assist them in coping with the terminal nature of her illness? Can they possibly help in other ways?
- What services will Mrs. Wise and her family most benefit from as her disease progresses?
- How can the needs of the family, including the grandchildren, best be met?
- Are there services that could be delivered via telehealth?
- How can the team collaborate in such a way that services are delivered seamlessly, and with as little disruption as possible to the family?

CASE

8.3

PROJECT: Task force to establish a new outreach program

PURPOSE: Homeless outreach service

SETTING: Grant-funded city agency

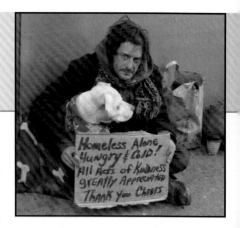

Your agency is one of the partners that was just awarded a large grant to establish a new homeless outreach program in the large city where you live. You have been asked by your director to join the team that will be developing the program. You have experience working with nonprofit health service programs, and you work well with people from diverse backgrounds. The other people on the team represent a variety of different disciplines. It is likely that some of you will continue to work with the program once it is established, but at this time it is not even clear what services will be needed.

There are certain aspects of the program that are dictated by the grant's sponsors. Part of the grant will be used to refurbish a one-block-long row of two-storey homes donated by the city that is located in a blighted area designated for urban renewal. Medical support will be provided through a program that pays off medical student loans if the new graduate works at least 2 years in designated areas of need or with underserved populations, such as the homeless. This sponsor is waiting to hear from the development team so they know how many physicians and/or physician extenders (physician assistants and nurse practitioners) to recruit for this program. A separate grant that was awarded with this program is targeted to women's health services for low-income women. Another condition of the grant is that it must include a service for individuals with drug and alcohol addiction. Your understanding is that this is expected to be similar to a methadone clinic; however, naltrexone has largely replaced methadone. Another additional small grant will be awarded if your team decides to incorporate acupuncture into the drug and alcohol treatment program. A final service that will be included is a vocational rehabilitation program.

The tasks that your team will be working on are as follows:

1. Identify the different services that the homeless outreach program will provide.
2. Identify what related services already exist in the area that you need to coordinate with, such as shelters, food kitchens, etc.
3. Clarify how you will reach the target population to bring them into your services–will it be different for each service?
4. What space needs will each service have? Can some services share space? What services can use the second-storey space?
5. How do you integrate the program into the neighborhood so that you are viewed as a "good neighbor?"
6. What staffing will you need for the different services? Can some staff be shared between services? What hours will each be open?
7. Will clients always need to get to you to receive services, or will you take some of the services to them?

8. How will the professionals coordinate their services and communication so that the client can seamlessly receive a variety of services from you?

9. What strategic outcomes need to be tracked to document the success of your program?

CASE

8.4

CLIENT: Albert Kirschoff, 68-year-old Ukrainian male

CONDITION: Diabetes with blindness and above-knee amputation

SETTING: Outpatient diabetes clinic

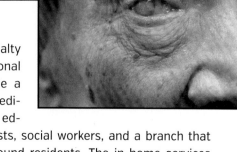

You and the rest of your team work at a specialty diabetes clinic that is affiliated with the regional medical center. Services in the clinic include a wound clinic, a prosthetic service, internal medi- cine services, nutrition counseling and nurse ed- ucators, vision experts, podiatrists, neurologists, social workers, and a branch that provides some in-home services for home-bound residents. The in-home services include skilled nursing and physical and occupational therapy. You are proud of the positive impact you are able to have on your clients' lives in the face of this serious disease.

Albert Kirschoff is a new client at the clinic. From his medical record you see that he is 68 years old, and was diagnosed with type II diabetes when he was 48. He has Social Security Disability Insurance and Medicare Part A and Part B. He and his fam- ily own a delicatessen in the city, and he was used to working long days. He immi- grated to the United States as a teenager from the Ukraine. He met his wife, Lydia, on the ship that he arrived on, and married her when they were both 18. They have one daughter, Mia, who lives nearby with her husband, and helps with the store. Mr. and Mrs. Kirschoff live in a two-bedroom apartment above the delicatessen. He still goes down to the store every day and drinks coffee at the corner table and advises his wife and daughter as well as the rest of the staff on running the business. He has a few friends from the neighborhood who join him in the afternoon.

Ever since he was first diagnosed, Mr. Kirschoff has had a great deal of difficulty learning to regulate his blood sugar levels. As a result, he began having serious com- plications from the disease by age 60. He has lost most of the vision in both eyes, and has had an above-knee amputation of his left leg. He has learned to walk with a pros- thesis, but since receiving it he has lost a significant amount of weight. Unfortunately, the weight loss affected the fit of the prosthesis and he developed a pressure ulcer on his residual limb. This open area has not healed well, and the infection has now spread to the nearby femur, resulting in osteomyelitis. Mr. Kirschoff was hospitalized last week, when a peripherally inserted central venous catheter (PICC line) was placed, through which he is receiving Vancomycin 1 g daily. He will need weekly bloodwork to monitor Vancomycin levels and kidney function. The surgeon who had previously per- formed the amputation recommended vacuum-assisted closure to improve the heal- ing. The wound vacuum consists of a sponge that is cut to the size and shape of the wound, placed in the wound bed, and covered with an occlusive dressing. It then has a suction disk attached which is connected to a portable vacuum pump. This draws out any drainage, keeps the wound bed moist while protecting the surrounding skin, and encourages granulation of the wound bed.

Mr. Kirschoff did not want to stay in the hospital any longer and talked to his phy- sician about support services in the community. Due to his multiple complications, his attending physician has referred Mr. Kirschoff to your clinic, where he and his family will benefit from the many services you offer. His medications include: Lantus insulin 50 units administered subcutaneously (SQ) every evening, plus Novolog insulin sliding scale based on blood sugar level before each meal, and Vicodin 5/325 (5 mg hydrocodone and 325 mg Tylenol) 1 to 2 tablets every 6 hours as needed for pain.

Questions as You Begin

Consider these questions as you begin developing this case:

- What is the most important factor in Mr. Kirschoff's quality of life?
- Can his living quarters be modified or moved so that he can more easily get around, without losing access to the family business?
- Until the wound vacuum is finished and his pressure ulcer is healed so that he can wear his new prosthesis, should he avoid going into the deli restaurant?
- What is the best way to support him in gaining better control over his blood sugar levels?

REFERENCES

1. American Occupational Therapy Association. The role of occupational therapy in primary care. 2014. http://www.aota.org/-/media/Corporate/Files/Publications/Primary-Care-Position-Paper.PDF.
2. American Occupational Therapy Association. Occupational therapy in primary care: an emerging area of practice. AOTA LEARN Continuing Education Article CEA0814. *OT Practice*. 2014;19(15).
3. Pellegrino E. Interdisciplinary education in the health professions: assumptions, definitions, and some notes in teams. Educating for the health team. Conference report of the Institute of Medicine. Washington, DC: National Academies Press; 1972.
4. Berwick E, Nolan T, Whittington J. The triple aim: care, health and cost. *Health Aff*. 2008;27:759–769. http://dx.doi.org/10.1377/hlthaff.27.3.759.
5. American Occupational Therapy Association. 2011 Accreditation Council for Occupational Therapy Education (ACOTE®) Standards and Interpretive Guide (effective July 31, 2013). 2011. http://www.aota.org/-/media/Corporate/Files/EducationCareers/Accredit/StandardsReview/guide/2011-Standards-and-Interpretive-Guide.ashx.

Student Skills Assessment

CLINICAL SKILLS SELF-ASSESSMENT: PRE-SURVEY

Name: _____ Date: _____

This survey is designed to help you evaluate your treatment and clinical reasoning skills as you prepare to enter the field of occupational therapy. The resulting scores will allow you to create a personal development plan and select cases from this text that will best fit your plan.

Part I: Treatment Conditions

A. Overall, how well prepared do you feel right now to evaluate and treat clients with typical diagnoses that you have studied?

1   2   3   4   5   6   7   8   9   10

I would not be capable of   *I feel very confident that I could*
providing any effective OT   *provide effective OT*
evaluation or treatment   *evaluation and treatment*

B. Please enter a score between 1 (very low) and 10 (very high) for each category below that reflects your perception of your ability to successfully identify and administer assessments and interventions for clients with typical diagnoses.

    1. Traumatic and repetitive stress musculoskeletal conditions
       (e.g., carpal tunnel syndrome, arm fractures, tendon repairs)   _____
    2. Chronic musculoskeletal conditions (e.g., rheumatoid arthritis)   _____
    3. Traumatic neurological injuries (e.g., cerebral vascular accident, spinal cord injury) _____
    4. Progressive neurological conditions (e.g., multiple sclerosis, dementia) _____
    5. Cardiopulmonary conditions
       (e.g., myocardial infarction, chronic obstructive pulmonary disease) _____
    6. Organ system conditions (e.g., burns, diabetes, cancer)   _____
    7. Mental disorders (e.g., major depression, schizophrenia)   _____

C. Why do you think your highest scores above are this high?

D. Please list 3–5 reasons that you think your lowest scores above are this low:

E. Personal Development Plan:

Based on your insights from C and D above, answer the following questions:

1. What type of diagnoses would you most benefit from working on?

2. What learning strategies have worked best for you in the past?

3. What do you need to do outside of class to reinforce your learning?

Part II: Practice Settings

A. Occupational therapy is delivered in a variety of traditional and nontraditional practice settings. The different environments influence the resources you have for treatment including space, equipment and time. Different settings may have different team members working alongside the OT, requiring you to adjust your focus.

Overall, how well prepared do you feel right now to evaluate and treat clients in a variety of different practice settings?

1   2   3   4   5   6   7   8   9   10

I feel prepared to treat   *I feel very confident that I could*
in very few different settings   *treat in a wide variety*
                                                        of practice settings

B. In each area below, please enter a number between 1 (very low) and 10 (very high) that reflects your perception of your ability to adjust your treatment to the demands of each practice setting.

1. Acute care inpatient (medical)	_____
2. Inpatient mental health	_____
3. Inpatient rehabilitation facility (IRF)	_____
4. Skilled nursing facility	_____
5. Intermediate care facility (ICF)	_____
6. Home health	_____
7. Outpatient (medical)	_____
8. Day treatment (medical or social model)	_____
9. School-based	_____
10. Worksite therapy	_____

C. Why do you think your highest scores above are this high?

D. Please list 3–5 reasons why you think your lowest scores above are this low:

E. Personal Development Plan:

Based on your insights from C and D above, answer the following questions:
1. What type of practice setting would you most benefit from working on?

2. What learning strategies do you think would be most helpful to your acquiring these skills?

3. What do you need to do outside of class to reinforce your learning?

Part III: Clinical Reasoning Skills
A. Clinical reasoning is not only about making treatment decisions based on best practice. It is also about developing client-centered treatment plans, modifying the plan based on conditions and response to treatment, as well as the ability to develop a therapeutic relationship with diverse clients.

Overall, how strong do you feel your clinical reasoning skills are right now?

| | 1 | 2 | 3 | 4 | 5 | 6 | 7 | 8 | 9 | 10 |

*I feel I have very weak
clinical reasoning skills*

*I feel I have very strong
clinical reasoning skills*

B. Please rate yourself between 1 (very low) and 10 (very high) in the following areas:

1. Ability to identify the critical areas and client needs that should be addressed in an intervention plan   _____
2. Ability to observe a client's behavior and identify important clinical information   _____
3. Ability to develop client-centered occupational performance goals for a client   _____
4. Ability to grade activities and modify plans to make adjustments based on a client's performance   _____
5. Ability to develop a home exercise/activity plan for the client   _____
6. Ability to understand and modify your approach and plans based on a client's unique context (social, economic, cultural, etc.)   _____
7. Ability to use a variety of interactive strategies effectively (Therapeutic Use of Self)   _____

C. Why do you think your highest scores above are this high?

D. Please list 3–5 reasons that you think your lowest scores are this low:

E. Personal Development Plan:

Based on your insights from C and D above, answer the following questions:

1. What type of clinical reasoning skills would you most benefit from working on?

2. What learning strategies do you think would be most helpful to your acquiring these skills?

3. What do you need to do outside of class to reinforce your learning?

Thank you for your thoughtful assessment.

CLINICAL SKILLS SELF-ASSESSMENT: POST-SURVEY

Name: _____ Date: _____

This survey is designed to help you re-evaluate your treatment and clinical reasoning skills after using this text. The resulting scores will assess your progress, and assist you in planning for continuing development.

Part I: Treatment Conditions

A. Overall, how well prepared do you feel right now to evaluate and treat clients with typical diagnoses that you have studied?

1   2   3   4   5   6   7   8   9   10

I would not be capable of   *I feel very confident that I could*
providing effective OT evaluation   *provide effective evaluation*
or treatment   *and treatment*

B. Please enter a score between 1 (very low) and 10 (very high) for each category below that reflects your perception of your ability to successfully identify and administer assessments and interventions for clients with typical diagnoses.

1. Traumatic and repetitive stress musculoskeletal conditions
   (e.g., carpal tunnel syndrome, arm fractures, tendon repairs) _____
2. Chronic musculoskeletal conditions (e.g., rheumatoid arthritis) _____
3. Traumatic neurological injuries (e.g., cerebral vascular accident, spinal cord injury) _____
4. Progressive neurological conditions (e.g., multiple sclerosis, dementia) _____
5. Cardiopulmonary conditions
   (e.g., myocardial infarct, chronic obstructive pulmonary disease) _____
6. Organ system conditions (e.g., burns, diabetes, cancer) _____
7. Mental disorders (e.g., major depression, schizophrenia) _____

C. What do you think contributed most to your scores above that improved?

D. Please list 3–5 reasons why you think your lowest scores above are still this low:

Part II: Practice Settings

A. Occupational therapy is delivered in a variety of traditional and nontraditional practice settings. The different environments influence the resources you have for treatment including space, equipment and time. Different practice settings may have different team members working alongside the OT, requiring you to adjust your focus.

How well prepared do you feel right now to evaluate and treat clients in a variety of different practice settings?

1   2   3   4   5   6   7   8   9   10

I feel prepared to treat in very few   *I feel very confident that I could*
different settings   *treat in a wide variety of settings*

B. In each area below, please enter a number between 1 (very low) and 10 (very high) that reflects your perception of your ability to adjust your treatment to the demands of each practice setting.

1. Acute care inpatient (medical)   _____
2. Inpatient mental health   _____
3. Inpatient rehabilitation facility (IRF)   _____
4. Skilled nursing facility   _____
5. Intermediate care facility (ICF)   _____
6. Home health   _____
7. Outpatient (medical)   _____
8. Day treatment (medical or social model)   _____
9. School-based   _____
10. Worksite therapy   _____

C. What do you think contributed most to your scores above that improved?

D. Please list 3–5 reasons why you think your lowest scores above are still this low:

Part III: Clinical Reasoning Skills

A. Clinical reasoning is not only about making treatment decisions based on best practice. It is also about developing client-centered treatment plans, modifying the plan based on conditions and response to treatment, as well as the ability to develop a therapeutic relationship with diverse clients.

Overall, how strong do you feel your clinical reasoning skills are right now?

     1   2   3   4   5   6   7   8   9   10

I feel I have very weak clinical   *I feel I have very strong clinical*
reasoning skills   *reasoning skills*

B. Please rate yourself between 1 (very low) and 10 (very high) in the following areas:

1. Ability to identify the critical areas and client needs that should be addressed in an intervention plan   _____
2. Ability to observe a client's behavior and identify important clinical information   _____
3. Ability to develop client-centered occupational performance goals for a client   _____
4. Ability to grade activities and modify plans to make adjustments based on a client's performance   _____
5. Ability to develop a home exercise/activity plan for the client   _____
6. Ability to understand and modify your approach and plans based on a client's unique context (social, economic, cultural, etc.)   _____
7. Ability to use a variety of interactive strategies effectively (Therapeutic Use of Self)   _____

C. What do you think contributed most to your scores above that improved?

D. Please list 3–5 reasons that you think your lowest scores are still low:

Part IV: Personal Development Plan

A. Please review the Personal Development Plan you created in the pre-survey at the start of this manual.

How well did you carry out your Personal Development Plan?

1	2	3	4	5	6	7	8	9	10

I carried out very little of the Personal Development Plan I created

I was very effective in carrying out my Personal Development Plan

B. Please explain your score in IV. A. above.

C. Professional development is an ongoing process. Regardless of what area of practice you ultimately work in, therapists must apply a broad field of knowledge not only to pass the NBCOT exam, but throughout your professional career in occupational therapy. What do you think you need to do going forward to improve your skills in the areas that remain low? Use as much space as you need. Be as specific and detailed as possible.

Thank you for your thoughtful assessment.

Case Development Protocol: Steps at a Glance

Step 1. What demographic information do I have for my client?

1. Review your case and list the basic demographic information.
2. What other basic information do you need that is not in the case description? What other source(s) might supply this information?

Step 2. What information can I find about my client's primary condition?

1. Review your case and document the primary condition or diagnosis you will be treating. Include any mention of symptoms, and any objective data about the condition or diagnosis.
2. Is all of the information you found relevant to your occupational therapy treatment? Explain your answer.
3. What type(s) of clinical reasoning did you use to guide your answer to question 2?

Step 3. Does my client have any secondary conditions?

1. Review your case and identify any secondary conditions, complications, or comorbidities.
2. Will the client's secondary condition affect your treatment of the primary condition? Explain your answer.

Step 4. What information can I find to help expand my awareness of my client as a whole person, more than just a diagnosis?

1. Review your case and identify any information related to personal context.
2. Next to each piece of information note what aspect of the person's life it relates to (e.g., support network, cultural affiliation, education, work status, financial status, and so on).

Step 5. Who else will be on the interprofessional team?

1. Consider the setting in which you will be "treating" and the condition to be addressed for your case.
2. Review your case and list all disciplines that are likely to be working with this client.

Step 6. What is the preliminary plan for my client after discharge?

1. Review your case to find any information related to anticipated length of stay, expected outcomes of care, and preliminary discharge plans.
2. Make note of this information for later consideration when you prepare your discharge summary.

Step 7. What questions do I ask my client when we first meet?

1. Review the basic demographic and personal context information from Steps 1 and 4. Create a list of interview questions you would like to ask your client to complete the occupational profile.
2. Use the Occupational Therapy Practice Framework-III (OTPF-III) to help you think of other areas you may have overlooked that could be important to your client. Add questions from this review to your list of interview questions.
3. Comment on the techniques you will use during the interview to gain your client's trust and develop a therapeutic relationship. (In other words, how will you employ Therapeutic Use of Self and interactive reasoning?)
4. What type of clinical reasoning influenced you in developing your list of initial interview questions?

Step 8. How do I develop the occupational profile?

1. Jot down notes about the client's likely answers to your interview questions from Step 7. Using your interactive reasoning skill, try to appreciate the individual's lived experience, including the illness experience.
2. Using the demographic and other background information from your previous case review as well as your projected answers to the interview questions, develop a 1- to 2-page occupational profile of your client. Make sure to include all relevant areas from the discussion above about what is included in an occupational profile. Refer to this profile throughout the remainder of your case, as it will represent your client.

Step 9. How will my client's occupational profile affect treatment?

1. Referring to the profile you developed in Step 8, discuss the implications for occupational therapy treatment by answering this question: "Now that I know the

information from my client's occupational profile, what types of modifications will I need to make to my assessments, interventions, or treatment approach?"

Step 10. How do I prepare for evidence-based practice?

1. Review academic and other scholarly sources to familiarize yourself with your client's primary condition. Compare the information you find to that supplied in your case to determine which specific symptoms your client displays.
2. Review scholarly sources for up-to-date evidence-based treatment information. Summarize your findings. What do you think about these findings? Are the results generalizable to this setting and this client? How does this information guide you or inform your occupational therapy treatment choices?
3. List preliminary ideas for assessments you might administer to your client.
4. What type(s) of clinical reasoning did you use in creating your list for question 3?
5. What preliminary thoughts do you have about a conceptual practice model that might work well for clients who have this primary condition? Explain.

Step 11. What effect will the primary and secondary condition(s) have on my client?

1. Using the occupational profile you created in Step 8 and your knowledge of your client's health condition(s) from Steps 2 and 3, describe the impact of the primary and secondary conditions on your client's activities of daily living (ADLs), instrumental activities of daily living (IADLs), work, play, and leisure.
2. Describe the illness experience for your client. What do you anticipate your client's attitude will be concerning his or her condition?
3. Describe the likely impact of the primary and secondary condition(s) on your client's future goals.
4. What type of clinical reasoning did you use to answer questions 2 and 3?

Step 12. What do you anticipate the treatment environment will be like?

1. Describe in detail the likely physical treatment space for your case.
2. Describe the impact of the physical space on your treatment: what pragmatic decisions will you need to make to use the space you have most effectively?
3. Describe the types of equipment and supplies you will most likely have available to you in this setting.

Step 13. How long will I be able to treat my client?

1. Estimate the average length of stay (LOS) for your setting for a person with the same condition as your client.
2. Describe how long your treatment sessions will likely be and how frequently they will occur (e.g., once a week in a 1-hour group session; once a week for a half-hour private session).

3. Using pragmatic reasoning, describe how these time frames will affect your treatments. What adjustments or priorities will you need to make to ensure you use your therapy time with your client as effectively as possible?

Step 14. What will my role be on the interprofessional team?

1. In Step 5, you identified the disciplines that will likely be on your client's interprofessional team. Now describe each discipline's major focus with your client, including occupational therapy in the list.
2. What effect, if any, do you think the other disciplines on your client's team will have on your OT focus?

Step 15. What specific assessment tools will I use in the evaluation process with this client?

1. Using the information from Step 10, list each assessment tool or assessment process you want to use in evaluating your client. Next to the name of each tool, identify what the tool is used to measure. Review Steps 10 and 11 to make sure you are including an assessment of all relevant factors that underlie occupational performance, including client factors, performance skills, and performance patterns.
2. Note how much time you think will be needed to administer each assessment, and add up the total time. Compare this time to the amount of time you will have available in one to two treatment sessions. If necessary, prioritize and revise your list.
3. Do your choices of assessment tools fit with the conceptual practice model you suggested using in Step 10? If not, how will you resolve this conflict?
4. List other tools or processes you considered but did not choose. Explain your clinical reasoning for each.

Step 16. What will the results be from my assessments?

1. Print a copy of the score sheet for each assessment you will use. If it is a nonstandardized observational assessment, create a form to capture your observations. (Tip: Think of the symptoms your client demonstrates, and typical symptoms for this condition.)
2. Review your documentation of the primary condition's symptoms from Step 2, the occupational profile from Step 8, and your description of the impact of the condition on your client's performance from Step 11; then, complete the assessment forms. Use your understanding of the client's condition to make logical assumptions about what results you might see for someone with this condition. Score each standardized form.
3. In paragraph form, briefly summarize your professional findings from the assessments. This brief, professional summary will help the other disciplines on the care team understand the results of your occupational therapy assessment.

Step 17. How do I begin an intervention plan?

1. Using the OTPF-III worksheet in Appendix D, place checkmarks in the boxes next to the categories that you believe are relevant (R), somewhat relevant (SR), or not relevant (NA) for your case. For each item marked relevant, note in the comment section to the right what the implications are—i.e., how does this occupation, client factor, or performance skill apply to this case? Check as relevant only those areas on which you think OT would focus in this setting.
2. Using the Intervention Plan form in Appendix E and your previous demographic information, fill in your client's identifying information at the top of the form.

Step 18. What areas should I focus on in treatment?

1. Review the list of your client's symptoms from Step 10 and their impact on performance from Step 11, and create a bulleted list of your client's deficits in occupational performance. Add the list to the OT Intervention Plan.
2. Review your list and revise as needed to make sure it reflects problems that are:
   - related to the condition for which the client was referred;
   - appropriate for OT to address within the given treatment setting and team;
   - reasonable to address within the expected time frame of treatment; and
   - meaningful to your client.
3. Review the OTPF-III with your client in mind. Does this review give you additional ideas about areas that you should address? Are you using "OT language" in your list? Make any necessary adjustments to your list of performance deficits on the Intervention Plan.

Step 19. What are my client's strengths?

1. Review the occupational profile you created in Step 8. Make a bulleted list of your client's strengths and add them to the Intervention Plan.
2. Review the OTPF-III with your client in mind. Does this review give you additional ideas about areas of strength that you might be able to use in therapy? Are you using "OT language" in your list? Make any necessary adjustments to the Intervention Plan's list of your client's strengths.

Step 20. What occupational performance goals will my client and I be working toward?

1. Create three to five long-term occupational performance goals for your client, and add them to your Intervention Plan.
2. For each long-term goal, write one or two short-term goals and add them to your Intervention Plan.

Step 21. What types of interventions will I use with my client?

1. List on your Intervention Plan the general types of interventions you plan to use. Include passive and active interventions, preparatory activities, and patient education activities.
2. Do your choices of interventions fit with the conceptual practice model you suggested using in Step 10? If not, how will you resolve this conflict? Explain.

Step 22. How frequently will I treat my client?

1. Complete the frequency and estimated length of treatment portion of your Intervention Plan.
2. Sign and initial your Intervention Plan with your professional initials.

Step 23 How will my first five treatment sessions be organized?

1. At the top of each column on the 5-Day Treatment Session Planning Template in Appendix D, fill in the estimated treatment time you will have on each date of service for the setting in your case.
2. Enter the name of the assessment(s) you plan to administer on the first day of treatment. Add the approximate amount of time it will take you to administer next to each.
3. Add assessment(s) to the Plan section at the bottom of the first day, to show what you will do on the second day of treatment.
4. Continue adding assessments as needed for the remaining days. Include any reassessments that are likely to take place in the first 5 days of treatment.
5. Add specific interventions to the first day of the 5-Day Treatment Session Planning Template.
6. In the Plan section at the bottom, make suggestions for what you will work on the next day.
7. Continue filling in interventions for the remaining days.
8. Review your plan. Are all occupational performance goals from the Intervention Plan addressed in the first 5 days? What adjustments would improve your plan? In your case development report, comment on changes or improvements you decided to make to your first draft of the 5-Day Treatment Session Planning Template.
9. What guided you in making these improvements? What type(s) of clinical reasoning did you use?

Step 24. What "home program" would best support my client's progress?

1. Add your home program plans to the bottom of the 5-Day Treatment Session Planning Template for each day. Make sure to consider how the client's home

environment, social supports, and financial resources might affect the home program.

2. Create handouts to give your client to support his or her progress toward occupational performance goals.

Step 25. How will I communicate my daily treatment activity?

1. From Appendix E, use the Daily Treatment Note form to prepare one daily note for each of the first 5 days of treatment for your case.

Step 26. What discharge plan does my client need?

1. From Appendix E, use the Discharge Planning Template to complete a discharge plan for your client.
2. Describe any challenges you encountered in developing a discharge plan for your client. Did you need to make any assumptions about your client's support system, resources, or personal context?
3. What type(s) of clinical reasoning did you use in developing the discharge plan? Explain.
4. Create any necessary handouts that will help your client after he or she is discharged. This might include contact information that would be needed in the event of problems, or community resources to support ongoing recovery.
5. Make sure your plan takes into account any relevant secondary conditions.

Step 27. How can an occupational therapy assistant and an occupational therapist work together most effectively to coordinate the OT services for my client?

1. Consider the setting you are working in and your client's condition. Review your first five treatment sessions. Describe which tasks and activities you would have an occupational therapy assistant do, and which you would have an occupational therapist do.
2. Explain your reasoning. Consider conditional, procedural, and ethical reasoning.

Step 28. How will I address ethical issues as I provide care?

1. Review the section on ethical reasoning in Chapter 1 of this book, "Informing Your Clinical Choices."
2. Next, review your case and identify any ethical issues you anticipate a possible need to address as you work with your client.
3. Using your interactive reasoning and TUOS skills, describe how you will address any ethical issues you have identified.

Index of Conditions by Practice Setting

Inpatient Treatment Settings

Critical Care Hospital Units

1. Acquired brain injury (Case 4.1, p. 94)
2. Burns to hands and face (Case 6.2, p. 144)

Medical and Surgical Units

1. Fractured humerus with ORIF (Case 3.2, p. 66)
2. Upper extremity amputation (Case 3.3, p. 69)
3. Flexor tendon repair (Case 3.6, p. 77)
4. Total hip replacement (Case 3.7, p. 80)
5. Left cerebrovascular accident (Case 4.2, p. 97)
6. Various conditions (Case 8.1, p. 163)

Cardiopulmonary Units

1. Myocardial infarction with CABG (Case 5.1, p. 130)
2. AIDS-related pneumonia (Case 5.2, p. 132)
3. Congestive heart failure (Case 5.4, p. 138)

Inpatient Rehabilitation Facility (IRF)

1. Acquired brain injury (Case 4.1, p. 94)
2. Right cerebral vascular accident (Case 4.3, p. 100)
3. Spinal cord injury (Case 4.5, p. 107)

Transitional Care/Short-Term Rehabilitation

1. Fractured humerus with ORIF (Case 3.2, p. 66)
2. Left cerebral vascular accident (Case 4.2, p. 97)

Inpatient Mental Health Facility

1. Major depressive disorder with suicidal ideation (Case 7.1, p. 152)
2. Posttraumatic stress disorder with alcohol abuse (Case 7.4, p. 158)

Community-Based Outpatient Treatment Settings

Outpatient Rehabilitation Clinic

1. Carpal tunnel syndrome with release (Case 3.1, p. 64)
2. Upper extremity amputation (Case 3.3, p. 69)
3. Lateral epicondylitis (Case 3.4, p. 73)
4. Colles fracture with ORIF (Case 3.5, p. 75)
5. Flexor tendon repair (Case 3.6, p. 77)
6. Rheumatoid arthritis (Case 3.8, p. 83)
7. Trigger finger release (Case 3.9, p. 86)
8. Dupuytren's contracture (Case 3.10, p. 88)
9. Low back pain (herniation between L5 and S1) (Case 3.11, p. 90)
10. Radial nerve injury (Case 4.4, p. 105)
11. Parkinson's disease (Case 4.8, p. 116)
12. Cancer with mastectomy and lymphedema (Case 6.4, p. 148)

Specialty Outpatient Clinics

1. Type 1 diabetes with renal failure (Case 6.3, p. 146)
2. Low vision (open-angle glaucoma) (Case 6.1, p. 142)
3. Diabetes with blindness and above-knee amputation (Case 8.4, p. 172)

Community Mental Health Services

1. Paranoid schizophrenia with psychosis (Case 7.3, p. 156)
2. Homeless outreach service (Case 8.3, p. 170)

Day Treatment Settings

1. Multiple sclerosis (Case 4.6, p. 111)
2. Alzheimer's dementia (Case 4.9, p. 118)
3. Bipolar disorder with manic episode (Case 7.2, p. 154)

School-Based Services

1. Spina bifida (Case 4.10, p. 123)

In-Home Care

Homecare Agency

1. Rheumatoid arthritis (Case 3.8, p. 83)
2. Right cerebrovascular accident (Case 4.3, p. 100)
3. Spinal cord injury (Case 4.5, p. 107)
4. Muscular dystrophy (Case 4.7, p. 114)
5. Chronic obstructive pulmonary disease (Case 5.3, p. 136)

In-Home Hospice Care

1. Amyotrophic lateral sclerosis (Case 8.2, p. 168)

Residential Care Settings

Skilled Nursing Facility

1. Fractured humerus with ORIF (Case 3.2, p.67)
2. Multiple sclerosis (Case 4.6, p. 111)
3. Alzheimer's dementia (Case 4.9, p. 118)

Hospice Residence

1. AIDS-related pneumonia (Case 5.2, p. 132)

Intermediate Care Facility

1. Down syndrome (Case 4.11, p. 125)

Occupational Therapy Practice Framework Worksheet

Occupational Therapy Practice Framework Worksheet*

Category	Rating			Comments
	R	SR	N/A	
Table 1. Occupations				
Activities of Daily Living (ADLs)				
Bathing, showering				
Toileting and toilet hygiene				
Dressing				
Swallowing/eating				
Feeding				
Functional mobility				
Personal device care				
Personal hygiene and grooming				
Sexual activity				
Instrumental Activities of Daily Living (IADLs)				
Care of others (including selecting and supervising caregivers)				
Care of pets				
Child rearing				
Communication management				
Driving and community mobility				
Financial management				
Health management and maintenance				
Home establishment and management				
Meal preparation and cleanup				
Religious and spiritual activities and expression				
Safety and emergency maintenance				
Shopping				
Rest and Sleep				
Rest				
Sleep preparation				
Sleep participation				
Education				
Formal educational participation				
Informal personal educational needs or interests exploration (beyond formal education)				
Informal personal education participation				
Work				
Employment interests and pursuits				
Employment seeking and acquisition				
Job performance				
Retirement preparation and adjustment				
Volunteer exploration				
Volunteer participation				

Category	Rating			Comments
	R	SR	N/A	
Play				
Play exploration				
Play participation				
Leisure				
Leisure exploration				
Leisure participation				
Social Participation				
Community				
Family				
Peer, friend				
Table 2. Client Factors				
Values, Beliefs, and Spirituality				
Values				
Beliefs				
Spirituality				
Body Functions				
Mental functions				
Specific mental functions				
Global mental functions				
Sensory functions				
Neuromusculoskeletal and movement-related functions				
Muscle functions				
Movement functions				
Cardiovascular, hematological, immunological, and respiratory system functions				
Voice and speech functions; digestive, metabolic, and endocrine functions; genitourinary and reproductive functions				
Skin and related-structure functions				
Body Structures				
Structure of the nervous system				
Eyes, ears and related structures				
Structures involved in voice and speech				
Structures of the cardiovascular, immunological, and respiratory systems				
Structures related to the digestive, metabolic, and endocrine systems				
Structures related to the genitourinary and reproductive systems				
Structures related to movement				
Skin and related structures				
Table 3. Performance Skills				
Motor Skills				
Aligns				

Category	Rating			Comments
	R	**SR**	**N/A**	
Stabilizes				
Positions				
Reaches				
Bends				
Grips				
Manipulates				
Coordinates				
Moves				
Lifts				
Walks				
Transports				
Calibrates				
Flows				
Endures				
Paces				
Process Skills				
Paces				
Attends				
Heeds				
Chooses				
Uses				
Handles				
Inquires				
Initiates				
Continues				
Sequences				
Terminates				
Searches/locates				
Gathers				
Organizes				
Restores				
Navigates				
Notices/responds				
Adjusts				
Accommodates				
Benefits				
Social Interaction Skills				
Approaches/starts				
Concludes/disengages				
Produces speech				
Gesticulates				

Category	Rating			Comments
	R	**SR**	**N/A**	
Speaks fluently				
Turns toward				
Looks				
Places self				
Touches				
Regulates				
Questions				
Replies				
Discloses				
Expresses emotion				
Disagrees				
Thanks				
Transitions				
Times response				
Times duration				
Takes turns				
Matches language				
Clarifies				
Acknowledges and encourages				
Emphasizes				
Heeds				
Accommodates				
Benefits				
Table 4. Performance Patterns				
Person				
Habits				
Routines				
Rituals				
Roles				
Group or Population				
Routines				
Rituals				
Roles				
Table 5. Context and Environment				
Contexts				
Cultural				
Personal				
Temporal				
Virtual				
Environments				
Physical				

Category	Rating			Comments
	R	SR	N/A	
Social				
Table 6. Types of Occupational Therapy Interventions				
Occupations and Activities				
Occupations				
Activities				
Preparatory Methods and Tasks				
Preparatory Methods				
Splints				
Assistive technology and environmental modifications				
Wheeled mobility				
Preparatory tasks				
Education and Training				
Education				
Training				
Advocacy				
Advocacy				
Self-advocacy				
Group Interventions				
Groups				
Table 7. Activity and Occupational Demands				
Relevance and importance to client				
Objects used and their properties				
Space demands (related to the physical environment)				
Social demands (related to the social environment and virtual and cultural contexts)				
Sequencing and timing				
Required actions and performance skills				
Required body functions				
Required body structures				
Table 8. Approaches to Intervention				
Create, promote (health promotion)				
Establish, restore (remediation, restoration)				
Maintain				
Modify (compensation, adaptation)				
Prevent (disability prevention)				
Table 9. Outcomes				
Occupational performance				
Improvement				
Enhancement				
Prevention				

Category	Rating			Comments
	R	SR	N/A	
Health and wellness				
Quality of life				
Participation				
Role competence				
Well-being				
Occupational justice				

* Source: American Occupational Therapy Association. Occupational Therapy Practice Framework : Domain and Process. AOTA Press, 2014.
Used by permission.

Forms

DAILY TREATMENT NOTE (SOAP Format)

Patient Name: _____

OVERVIEW:

SUBJECTIVE:

OBJECTIVE:

ASSESSMENT:

PLAN:

Therapist signature: _____ **Date:** _____

5-DAY TREATMENT SESSION PLANNING TEMPLATE
INPATIENT REHABILITATION FACILITY

Patient Name: _____

Day 1	Day 2	Day 3	Day 4	Day 5
Assessments:	Assessments:	Assessments:	Assessments:	Assessments:
Interventions:	Interventions:	Interventions:	Interventions:	Interventions:
Plan:	Plan:	Plan:	Plan:	Plan:
HP:	**HP:**	**HP:**	**HP:**	**HP:**

INTERVENTION PLAN

Patient Name: _____

OVERVIEW:

OCCUPATIONAL PERFORMANCE DEFICITS

STRENGTHS

OCCUPATIONAL PERFORMANCE GOALS

   LTG:

   STG:

   STG:

   STG:

   LTG:

   STG:

   STG:

   STG:

GENERAL INTERVENTIONS

FREQUENCY:

Signature: _____   **Date:** _____

DISCHARGE PLAN

Patient Name: _____ **Identification number:** _____

Referring physician: _____

Date of admission: _____ Date of planned discharge: _____

Primary diagnosis: _____

Occupational performance at onset of therapy: _____

Long term occupational performace goals   **Goal status at discharge**

Comments on goals not achieved: _____
_____
_____

Potential safety issues at time of discharge: _____
_____
_____

Recommended placement after discharge: _____
_____
_____

Recommended referrals after discharge: _____
_____
_____

Therapist signature: _____ **Date of discharge summary:** _____

COMMUNITY-BASED THERAPEUTIC GROUP NOTES
Individual Group Note

Date: _____ **Name of Group:** _____ **Frequency of meetings:** _____

Number of Participants: _____

OBJECTIVE/OBSERVATIONS

Individual's appearance: (sloppy, neat, hygiene, grooming, revealing, conservative, mismatched, stylish)

Body language: (open and comfortable, tense and on-edge, guarded and closed)

Attention: (normal, inattentive, distractible, confused)

Mood, emotion expressed: (relaxed/ anxious, depressed/happy/hostile, labile/flat/euphoric, irritable)

Ability to express him/herself: (expressed self clearly and easily, had difficulty identifying emotions/needs, spoke over others/had difficulty stopping)

Interaction with other team members: (showed empathy, discussed meaningful personal issues, provided helpful feedback, attention-seeking, disruptive, not respectful of others)

Interaction with leader: Did you observe this individual taking risks? Was this reinforced/supported?

ASSESSMENT/INTERPRETATION

How did Group Leader try to meet this individual's needs?

How did other group members try to meet this individual's needs?

How did individual respond?

What role did this individual take in the group? (follower, initiator, energizer, information seeker, critique, encourager, harmonizer, gatekeeper)

APPLICATION/LEARNING

What insight did this individual gain from the session?

Were there other benefits to individual from group?

COMMUNITY-BASED THERAPEUTIC GROUP NOTES
General Group Process/Group Dynamics Note

Date: _____   **Name of Group:** _____   **Frequency of meetings:** _____

Number of Participants: _____   **Average length of attendance:** _____

OBJECTIVE/OBSERVATIONS

<u>Interaction between members</u>:

<u>Group process</u>:
Were ground rules obvious or referred to?

Did sharing and processing take place?

<u>Group dynamics</u>:
What roles did you observe individuals taking?

What problem behaviors did you observe?

ASSESSMENT/INTERPRETATION

What stage did this group appear to be in? (Use any theorist) Why?

APPLICATION/LEARNING

What learning did the group members take from this session?

COMMUNITY-BASED THERAPEUTIC GROUP NOTES
Group Leadership Note

Date: _____   Name of Group: _____   Frequency of meetings: _____

Number of Participants: _____   Closed or open group: _____   Average length of attendance: _____

Purpose of Group: _____

OBJECTIVE/OBSERVATIONS

How did the leader prepare for the group? (Introduction phase)

Leadership technique(s) observed:

Group response to technique(s):

Interaction between members & leader:
(Infrequent/prompted by leader, Frequent/some prompted by leader, Self initiated/spontaneous, hostile/territorial, friendly/comfortable, members primarily talked to leader)

What evidence did you see that this was a therapeutic and client-centered group?

ASSESSMENT/INTERPRETATION

What leadership style was being used?

What stage did this group appear to be in?

Did the leadership style complement the group needs?

APPLICATION/LEARNING

Was the purpose of the group achieved by most of the members?

Did the leader adjust his/her style in response to the group members and their needs?

Index

Note: Page numbers followed by "*f*" denote figures.